HEALTH ASSESSMENT

THROUGH THE LIFE SPAN

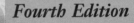 *Fourth Edition*

Mildred O. Hogstel, PhD, RN, C
Professor Emeritus
Harris School of Nursing
Texas Christian University
Fort Worth, Texas

Linda Cox Curry, PhD, RN
Professor
Harris School of Nursing
Texas Christian University
Fort Worth, Texas

 F. A. Davis Company • Philadelphia

F. A. Davis Company
1915 Arch Street
Philadelphia, PA 19103
www.fadavis.com

Printed in Canada

Last digit indicates print number: 10 9 8 7 6 5 4 3 2 1

Acquisitions Editor: Lisa B. Deitch
Developmental Editor: Danielle J. Barsky

As new scientific information becomes available through basic and clini
research, recommended treatments and drug therapies undergo changes. T
authors and publisher have done everything possible to make this book acc
rate, up to date, and in accord with accepted standards at the time of pul
cation. The authors, editors, and publisher are not responsible for errors
omissions or for consequences from application of the book, and make
warranty, expressed or implied, in regard to the contents of the book. A
practice described in this book should be applied by the reader in accordan
with professional standards of care used in regard to the unique circui
stances that may apply in each situation. The reader is advised always
check product information (package inserts) for changes and new informati
regarding dose and contraindications before administering any medicatio
Caution is especially urged when using new or infrequently ordered medic
tions.

Library of Congress Cataloging-in-Publication Data

Hogstel, Mildred O.
 Health assessment through the life span / Mildred O. Hogstel, Linda C
Curry.— 4th ed.
 p. ; cm.
 Rev. ed. of: Practical guide to health assessment through the life span. 3
ed. c2001.
 Includes bibliographical references and index.
 ISBN 0-8036-1293-1 (alk. paper)
 1. Nursing assessment—Handbooks, manuals, etc. I. Curry, Linda.
Hogstel, Mildred O. Practical guide to health assessment through the li
span. III. Title.
 [DNLM: 1. Nursing Assessment—Handbooks. 2. Medical Histo
Taking—Handbooks. 3. Physical Examination—Handbooks. WY 49 H71
2005]
 RT48.H643 2005
 616.07'5—dc22

 20040634

To Our Families and Students

PREFACE

Health assessment is an essential component of the nursing process and includes the health history; psychosocial history; physical, functional, and mental status examinations; and cultural, family, and environmental assessments. The essential components of the assessment process may be completed in a few minutes in an emergency; at the other extreme assessment may take place over several weeks in the patient's home. Depending on priorities, the nurse has to use judgment in deciding which parts of the assessment are needed for a specific patient in a certain setting.

The purpose of this book is to provide nursing students and practicing nurses in all areas, including community settings, with a practical and easy-to-use reference to the major components, sequence, and methods of health assessment. It is assumed that the user of this book will have completed courses in anatomy and physiology and will have completed, or currently be enrolled in, a course in health assessment.

This book can easily be kept in a pocket until needed. When the nurse is ready to perform any part of the assessment, the book may be placed on a table near the patient's bed or chair. The book has been designed for easy reference. The fourth edition has been expanded to include more content that will be helpful in better understanding the assessment process. New areas include assessment of the use of alternative and complementary therapies; antepartum and intrapartum assessment; expanded coverage of communication skills, especially when communicating with patients of different ages, with different needs, and from different cultural backgrounds; family communication and assessment: variations in physical assessment based on various cultural differences; and a basic orientation to and expansion of physical assessment techniques. The equipment needed, sequence, and techniques for each system have also been expanded. The steps of what to assess in carrying out a physical examination of each body system are listed. It should be noted that some of the assessment techniques (for example, an internal gynecologic examination and a prostate examination) are included as essential components of a total assessment, but they will not be performed by the novice practitioner.

Normal and/or common findings and *significant deviations* from normal are included for each system. *Common* findings are those that are not considered *normal* because they do not occur in everyone but that rarely need referral (e.g., solar lentigo in older adults or cradle cap in infants). *Common* and *significant* findings that should be referred for follow-up are shown in color. A special section, clinical alert, is also in color. This section notes special instructions the nurse needs to be aware of during the assessment and/or concerns related to the findings such as immediate referral.

A few sample diagnostic tests are listed for each system. The nurse will refer the patient to a physician, advanced nurse practitioner (where appropriate), or other health-care provider, who may order and evaluate the diagnostic tests. Sample North American Nursing Diagnosis Association (NANDA) nursing diagnoses are also included for each system. These are not meant to be inclusive because nursing diagnoses are very individualized. However, the samples should guide the reader toward other possible diagnoses. These diagnoses should be helpful in preparing individual care plans after the assessment phase. Essential patient and family education, home health notes, a list of associated community agencies, and health and wellness content for each system also have been expanded or added. Content on obesity, an increasing problem for all ages, and other content on health and wellness have been added.

Perinatal, pediatric, and geriatric adaptations have been revised for each section of the health history, physical examination, and patient family education. Cultural adaptations and additions have been made, where appropriate. For each body system, a brief sample of how to document the physical findings is presented. Samples of primarily *normal* and some *common abnormal* findings are documented. *Significant deviations* from normal will need more detailed documentation. These samples are only a general guide because methods of documentation vary with the institution or agency format, the setting, and the patient's needs or status.

The appendixes contain selected sample history, mental status, functional assessment, and physical assessment forms, as well as other reference material that will be helpful in performing and documenting a complete health assessment. A glossary of the most commonly used abbreviations and terms in health assessment appears at the back of the book so that other references will not be needed for this information. Following this is a list of specific references used in each of the three sections of the book and other health assessment resources, which may be consulted for further reading.

The authors believe that nurses will find this assessment book a helpful, time-saving clinical guide while they are learning or becoming more skilled in health assessment techniques in the classroom or any clinical setting in which they assess patients.

Mildred O. Hogstel, PhD, RN, C
Linda Cox Curry, PhD, RN

Acknowledgments

The authors express their appreciation to the contributors for their helpful additions, and to Susan Moore, Executive Assistant, College of Health and Human Sciences, Texas Christian University, for typing the manuscript.

Contributors

Pediatric Adaptations by
Marinda Allender, RN, MSN
Instructor
Harris School of Nursing
Texas Christian University
Fort Worth, Texas

Geriatric Adaptations by
Barbara Harty, RN, MSN, GNPC
Internal Medicine
Division of Geriatrics
University of North Texas Health Science Center
Fort Worth, Texas

Sherry Reese, RN, MSN, FNP-C
Internal Medicine
Division of Geriatrics
University of North Texas Health Science Center
Fort Worth, Texas

Health and Wellness Adaptations by
Pamela Jean Frable, ND, RN
Assistant Professor
Harris School of Nursing
Texas Christian University
Fort Worth, Texas

Nutrition Adaptations by
Lyn Dart, PhD, RD, LD
Assistant Professor
Department of Nutritional Sciences
Texas Christian University
Fort Worth, Texas

Contents

Part 3   **Body Organ and System
Assessment**   **75**

APPENDICES

List of Figures

List of Tables

PART

The Patient Interview and Health History

CHAPTER 1

Overview of the Nursing Process

The profession of nursing is made up of many roles and activities. Several scholars and theorists have defined the profession of nursing, but the most commonly accepted definition is the one offered in 1980 by the American Nurses' Association (ANA): "the diagnosis and treatment of human responses to actual or potential health problems." This means that nurses care for people, as individuals or groups, who are reacting to actual health problems. Additionally, nurses attempt to prevent problems and promote maintenance in people who are healthy.

The framework for nursing practice is the *nursing process*, which is an organized problem-solving method. The nursing process was defined and refined in the 1950s to 1970s. It is made up of five sequential steps: assessment, diagnosis, planning, implementation, and evaluation. Through application of the nursing process, the nurse is able to deliver nursing care, for example, to diagnose and treat human responses to health problems.

The nursing process also provides a common language for nurses to use in any geographic area or specialty practice. The ANA developed its standards of care around the nursing process, and the licensing examination is structured to test knowledge of the five steps in the process. The focus of this text is on the first step of the nursing process, assessment. The steps are briefly explained in the next section.

Assessment is focused on the collection of information about the patient and the patient's problem(s) to lay a foundation for the remainder of the process. Data may be *subjective,* that is, perceived only by the patient, or it may be *objective;* that is, it can be validated by the nurse or other health-care professional. Examples of subjective data include nausea, pain, and feelings of worthlessness. Examples of objective data include vomiting, facial expressions, physical behaviors, and laboratory data. Subjective data are most often collected during the nursing history, usually an interview. Objective data may be observed at any time but are most often collected during the physical examination or review of the medical record for laboratory or other findings.

The second step is *nursing diagnosis* and consists of clustering and organizing the data gathered during assessment. The data that fit together into a diagnosis category are then labeled with a diagnosis that guides the remainder of the nursing process. The diagnosis not only organizes the data but also provides a fast and articulate description of the patient's problems or needs. These nursing diagnoses are widely available and are reviewed annually by the North American Nursing Diagnosis Association (NANDA). Refer to Appendix A for the most current list of nursing diagnoses.

The third step in the nursing process is *planning.* This step has several components, including (a) placing the diagnoses in priority order, (b) identifying outcome criteria to facilitate evaluation, (c) identifying the nursing interventions necessary to reach the outcomes, and (d) documenting this step in the appropriate place and manner for the institution or agency. Planning is accomplished with the help of the patient and family and is essential to the effective delivery of care.

Implementation is the fourth step in the process. Using the plan as a guide, the nurse carries out the plan and communicates with other staff and the patient. In this step, the nurse may be teaching a new parent how to bathe a baby, an older adult how to inject a medication, or a family member how to change a dressing on a surgical wound. This step also includes the documentation of care in the patient record.

The fifth and final step of the nursing process is *evaluation.* In this step, the nurse assesses the patient's progress toward the outcomes identified in the planning process. If revisions in the care plan are necessary, they should be instituted. If the outcome has been reached, the problem is resolved. The evaluation step generates new assessment data, and the process continues.

The nursing process can be illustrated in the care of a patient on the first day after abdominal surgery and the activities involved in only one problem. The nurse collects the following data during assessment: The patient is crying and asking for pain relief, there is an 8-inch surgical incision across her lower abdomen, the patient is restless and guarding the incision during movement, and the patient has had no pain medication for 6 hours. A diagnosis of acute pain would guide the nurse toward suggested interventions such as providing comfort measures, administering medications, and encouraging family support. The planning phase includes proposed interventions and such details as how much medication to give and how often it can be given. For example, after the patient experienced relief, the nurse would plan to teach about pain management, including the timing of medications. The planning phase also includes identifying outcome criteria to guide evaluation methods such as assessing the patient's ability to sleep or function, as well as asking the patient to describe the level of pain relief. The implementation phase is the administration of medications, positioning the patient with pillows under the abdomen, and teaching about pain. This step also includes documenting the assessment data, nursing actions, and responses of the patient in the record. The last step is evaluation. In this example, the nurse would assess the patient's pain relief by asking the patient to rank the level of pain, as well as observing the patient's behavior, as observed by the ability to sleep or a relaxed facial expression.

To be effective, the nursing process requires significant knowledge and skills. For example, the nurse should have an understanding of physiology, psychology, chemistry, and nutrition to identify obesity in an adolescent and develop a plan of care. The nurse should have adequate skills to conduct a thorough assessment, such as auscultating breath sounds or describing a skin lesion. Finally, the nurse should have psychomotor skills to carry out activities such as diapering a newborn or inserting an intravenous catheter.

The purpose of this text is to assist the nurse in developing and mastering the skills and knowledge associated with the assessment phase of the nursing process. These include communication and technical skills based on a broad background in the sciences and humanities.

CHAPTER

Communication Skills

Effective communication is an essential component of the total nursing process. How a nurse speaks to, listens to, looks at, responds to, and touches a person often determines how that person will share information, thoughts, and feelings and participate with the plan of care. Most patients can tell by the nurse's first contact and approach what kind of relationship is likely to develop. Patients can usually tell if nurses are interested in them by the way they speak, stand, or sit and listen, as well as what they say.

Attentive listening is one of the most important skills a nurse can develop. And, it is not as easy as it sounds. Attentive listening—hearing what the other person is saying and understanding the meaning of words, gestures, and mannerisms—during a 1-hour session with a patient can be much more tiring and difficult than speaking for an hour.

Effective Communication

Effective *communication* is essential for successfully *interviewing* the patient to obtain his or her health history:

- *Communication* may be defined as one's attempt to understand another person's point of view from his or her frame of reference.
- *Interviewing* may be defined as conversation directed by the nurse for the explicit purpose of seeking information from the patient. It includes the use of verbal and nonverbal behavior by the nurse to communicate with the patient.
- *Communication* is used in every intervention with the patient from the time of admission and the taking of a health history through discharge planning and teaching home health-care needs.

Effective communication, although often time consuming, can enhance nursing care and possibly prevent problems later. When nurses develop trusting and open relationships with patients early in their care, the patients are usually more open, more cooperative, and less likely to complain or be upset if everything does not go as planned later.

Purposes of Therapeutic Communication

The purposes of therapeutic communication are to

- Exchange ideas, information, and feelings.
- Understand another person's point of view.
- Understand another person's frame of reference.
- Assist in establishing the nurse-patient relationship.
- Effect change in nurse-patient situations.
- Disseminate information.
- Assist in clarifying problems.
- Help patients create new patterns for healing and wellness.

Aspects of Each Message

- What the sender wants to convey.
- What the sender conveys.
- What the receiver hears.
- What the receiver thought he or she heard.
- How the receiver interprets the message (see Fig. 2–1).

The aspects of each message are influenced by positive or

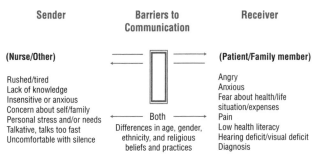

Sender	Barriers to Communication	Receiver
(Nurse/Other)		**(Patient/Family member)**
Rushed/tired		Angry
Lack of knowledge		Anxious
Insensitive or anxious		Fear about health/life
Concern about self/family		situation/expenses
Personal stress and/or needs	Both	Pain
Talkative, talks too fast	Differences in age, gender,	Low health literacy
Uncomfortable with silence	ethnicity, and religious	Hearing deficit/visual deficit
	beliefs and practices	Diagnosis

Figure 2-1 Components of communication.

negative factors that can affect the communication process. These include

- Individual qualities of each participant (beliefs, needs, values, sociocultural background, age, gender, and current physical and emotional status).
- Capacity of sender and receiver to speak and hear.
- Relationship between sender and receiver.
- Purpose of the communication.
- Content of message being sent.
- Setting and/or environmental conditions and distractions (setting may be unfamiliar to patient, which can cause anxiety).
- Previous experiences associated with the present situation.
- Language skill of interviewer.

Criteria for Effective Verbal Communication

- *Clarity:* Avoid ambiguous words and generalizations.
- *Simplicity:* Use lay terms and avoid medical terminology.
- *Timing and relevancy:* Send message when it needs to be sent in relation to the patient's interests and concerns.

REMEMBER

It is impossible not to communicate. When one is not using *verbal* communication, it must be remembered that *nonverbal* communication is occuring. Nonverbal communication is the exchange of messages without the use of words.

Nonverbal Communication

- Body language (e.g., use of hands or arms).
- Facial expressions.
- Eye contact (depends on culture).

- Lip movements.
- Gestures.
- Posture.
- Physical appearance (including clothes and grooming).
- Space (distance between two people).
- Touch (differentiate for skilled care and support).
- Silence (can be therapeutic or awkward).
- Qualities of voice (intonation, rate, rhythm, and pitch).
- Active listening.

Guidelines for Active and Effective Listening

- Avoid interruptions.
- Concentrate on the speaker.
- Maintain eye contact if culturally appropriate to do so.
- Lean toward and face the speaker.
- Maintain open posture, not crossed arms.
- Make a conscious effort to hear and *understand* the other person; avoid premature interpretations and judgments.
- Avoid extensive note taking.

Guidelines for Use of Touch

Touch is a form of nonverbal communication that is a learned behavior filled with meaning. Touch is generally not necessary in obtaining a health history but is necessary in performing a physical assessment. This poses a difficult problem for the nurse. In general, it is best to avoid the use of touch, particularly invasive procedures, until a nurse-patient relationship is well established and the nurse is knowledgeable about the beliefs related to touch in the particular culture. When touch becomes necessary, it is best used by members of the same gender and culture. If touch seems appropriate while taking a nursing history (e.g., if a patient should begin crying), gentle touch of the nurse's hand on the patient's upper arm or shoulder could be used.

■ Developmental Considerations in Communication

Age and gender are factors to consider when communicating with patients. The nurse does not communicate with a 5-year-old, a 45-year-old, or a 95-year-old in the same manner. Although the nurse should be himself or herself in each individual situation, variations in approach will be needed. For example, motherspeak (baby talk) is not appropriate past a certain age, and it should not be assumed that all 95-year-old people have a hearing deficit.

Infants

- Address the baby by given name.
- Do not address parents as "Mom" or "Dad."
- Speak to the infant before beginning assessment.

Toddlers

- Introduce yourself.
- Spend time talking to parent before approaching child.
- Allow parent to remain close to child.
- Have stuffed animal or toy for child to play with.
- Sit at eye level to child.

Preschoolers

- Introduce yourself.
- Call the child by name.
- Ask the child simple questions directly.
- Allow child to manipulate equipment before using it on child.
- Sit at eye level to child.

School-Age Children

- Address questions concerning habits and health promotion to the child.
- Encourage the child rather than the parent to answer.

- Provide explanations of assessment techniques as well as findings.
- Provide health teaching directly to the child.

Adolescents

- Obtain some preliminary history information from adolescent and parent.
- Ask to speak to adolescent alone.
- Discuss confidential issues with adolescent.
- Use open-ended questions ("Tell me about...." "Many teenagers are concerned about...").
- Listen and respond in a nonthreatening or non-judgmental manner.

Adults*

- Always face the person and establish eye contact.
- Speak slowly and clearly. Watch your accent.
- Always respect the rights and dignity of the person.
- Do not use complicated medical terminology.
- Use common lay terminology without being overly simplistic.
- Let the person set the pace of the conversation.
- Do not interrupt the person.
- Do not crowd the person unless you are invited or encouraged to come close.
- Avoid distracting body signals like finger tapping and seat shifting.
- Try not to appear distracted by unseemly or grotesque appearances or uncontrolled gestures.
- If you do not speak his or her language well, do not try at all, but get an interpreter or signer.
- Assume nothing.
- Sit if the person is sitting or lying down.

Source: Adapted from material provided by the Long-term Care Ombudsman Program of the Mental Health Association of Tarrant County.

- Always regard what the person has to say as important.
- Be kind and warm, but firm.
- Make no promises you cannot keep.
- Under some circumstances, silent presence can be very comforting and reassuring and can be a strong statement of concern and care.

Older Adults* (See also App. B)

PREPARATION

- Always introduce yourself by your full name and explain your role unless the person knows you by name or recognition.
- Never patronize an older person. Greet the person by Mr. Mrs., Ms., or Dr. and surname, unless the person asks you to use another name.
- Always respect the rights and dignity of the person.
- Do not make promises you cannot keep. Be honest and direct.
- Allow time to cultivate a trusting relationship.
- Let the person set the pace of the conversation. Fight the impulse to talk rather than listen.
- Always regard what the person has to say as important.
- Be dependable. Promise only what you can control.
- Be honest. Avoid giving false hope or stating platitudes.

GENERAL

- Identify yourself by name (do not be disappointed if some people forget). Repeat as needed.
- Call the person by the preferred name (use first name *only* if it is preferred).
- Avoid questions that can be answered with "yes" or "no."
- Avoid current slang and/or filler words (e.g., "you know; it's like, cool, man").

*Source: Written by Mildred O. Hogstel, Ph.D., R.N., C. (with suggestions from Ann Reban. M.S.N., R.N., C., Anne L. Lind. M.S.N., R.N., and Monnette Graves, M.S.N.).

- Keep yourself in the person's view so that he or she can see your face. (Talking at the side or in the back may cause difficulty with communication and confusion.)
- Use direct eye contact (unless the patient does not feel comfortable with that approach because of his or her culture). Sit or stand at the same level as the person.
- Use a calm, clear, slightly slower, lower-pitched voice. Do not speak loudly or shout because this can cause auditory discomfort.
- Speak louder only if you are sure the person has a hearing loss. (Check if you are uncertain.)
- Try not to sound angry if you must speak loudly.
- Repeat if necessary. Speak once the same way: if you are still not understood, rephrase.
- Eliminate background noise (e.g., television).
- Ask one question at a time and wait for a response.
- Allow time for responses. It may take a little longer than you expect.
- Do not interrupt the person because doing so discourages responses.
- *Listen attentively.*

WRITTEN

- Name tags with large type and category of personnel are helpful.
- Use written notes as reminders (e.g., names of family and friends).
- Label names of people on pictures.

BODY LANGUAGE

- Use an open, gentle approach and genuine smile.
- Use a gentle touch. (A gentle pat on the hand can test the person's response.)
- Evaluate acceptability of hugs. Response to touch and protection of personal space vary among individuals.
- A simple nod of the head is appropriate.

▣ Communicating With People Who Are Physically Challenged*

Communicating with People Who Are Hearing Impaired

- Find out if the person has a hearing aid.
- If the person wears a hearing aid and still has difficulty hearing, check to see if the hearing aid is in the person's ear, turned on, adjusted, and has a working battery.
- Wait until you are directly in front of the person, you have the person's attention, and you are close to the person before you begin speaking.
- Be sure that the person sees you as you approach her or him.
- Always face the person. Be on the same level with the person, whenever possible, and gain eye contact.
- Do not chew gum or smoke, and keep your hands away from your face while talking.
- Speak slowly and clearly.
- Do not let your voice trail or drop off at the end of a sentence or phrase.
- Never shout. Shouting distorts sound and turns word symbols into noise.
- Reduce background noises as much as possible when carrying on a conversation.
- Use simple, short sentences to make your conversation easier to understand.
- Do frequent checks to see if the person is understanding you.
- Write messages if necessary. Ask relatives how they communicate with the person.
- Do not be impatient. Allow ample time to converse with a hearing-impaired person. Being in a rush will compound everyone's stress and create barriers to having a meaningful conversation.

Source: Adapted from material provided by the Long-term Care Ombudsman Program of the Mental Health Association of Tarrant County.

Communicating with People Who Cannot Hear

Communicating with people who are deaf is similar to communicating with the hearing impaired.

- Ask relatives or friends of the person who cannot hear how they communicate.
- Write messages if the person can read.
- Use devices with illustrations (e.g., a picture board) to facilitate communication.
- Be concise with your statement and questions.
- Allow sufficient time to visit with the person.
- Face the person when speaking.
- If the person communicates with sign language, use interpreters qualified to interpret the type of sign language used.
- Communicating via a computer can be effective for people who are comfortable with technology.

Communicating with People Who Are Visually Impaired

- Touch is important. You might offer your hand or, if you are walking, offer use of your arm as guidance.
- Call out the person's name before touching. Touching lets a person know you are listening.
- Allow the person to touch you.
- Tell the person if you are leaving. Let the person know if others will remain in the room or if she or he will be alone.
- If you are in a group, always begin your comments by saying the name of the person to whom you are addressing.
- Treat the person who is visually impaired as you would an individual who is fully sighted. This will help the person you are talking with feel at ease and confident.
- Find out from the individual the extent of her or his impairment. Legal blindness is not necessarily total blindness.
- Use the words *see* and *look* normally.
- Explain what you are doing, as you are doing it.

- Encourage familiarity and independence whenever possible.
- Do not be overprotective.
- Be careful not to move things around in the room of a person who is visually impaired, unless the person asks you to move something.

Communicating with People Who Are Aphasic

Aphasia is a total or partial loss of the power to use or understand words. It is often the result of a stroke or other brain damage.

- Get the person's attention. Try to make sure there are no other distractions in the immediate area.
- Be patient, communicate only one idea at a time. and allow plenty of time. Speak slowly.
- Use simple, concrete adult language. Use short phrases.
- Be honest with the person. Do not pretend to understand a person when you do not.
- Allow the person who is aphasic to try to complete thoughts, to struggle with words. Avoid being too quick to guess what the person is trying to express.
- Encourage the person to write the word he or she is trying to use and read it out loud.
- Use of gestures or pointing to objects might be helpful.
- Use touch to aid in concentration, communication, reassurance, and encouragement, if appropriate.
- Pictures can be used with any patient who has experience or receptive deficit.

Communicating With People Who Are Cognitively Challenged

- Assess the individual's capacity to understand.
- Help the person to feel safe and secure.
- Ask simple yes or no questions. Speak slowly.
- Use positive statements. Help the person understand what you want him or her to do.

- If the person is having trouble communicating an idea, help with the word he or she is trying to find. Do not interrupt or appear impatient.
- Write down positive or reassuring information. Avoid giving information that may produce anxiety. Timing is important.
- Use short, clear, and concrete statements, one step at a time. Give step-by-step instructions.
- Clarify misspoken information given by the cognitively challenged individual.

Communicating With People Who Are Aggressive

- Speak softly. Be calm and reassuring.
- Avoid quick, sudden, or erratic movements.
- Never argue or try to reason with the person.
- Be empathetic.
- Keep out of striking distance.
- Never threaten verbally or strike back; this is abuse.
- Avoid cornering the person. Keep a clear pathway out of the room.

Cultural Variations in Communicating and Interviewing

When nurses communicate with patients from cultures different from their own, the likelihood of miscommunication increases dramatically. There are major problems in verbal communication; however, there are as many pitfalls, if not more, in nonverbal, transcultural communication.

General Guidelines for Transcultural Therapeutic Communication

- Maintain an open attitude.
- Speak in a clear, slow manner.
- RRS: Restate, reflect, and summarize.

- Write important information, using drawings and pictures to increase understanding.

Communicating with Patients with Limited English Proficiency (LEP)*

- Patients who cannot speak, read, or understand English at a level that permits effective interaction with clinical and non-clinical staff are considered LEP.
- In the absence of bilingual health-care providers who have sufficient language skills related to health-care issues, use medical interpreters (United States Department of Health and Human Services, Office of Minority Health. (March 2001)
- Speak directly to patients in English and allow patients to speak directly to you in their language. The interpreters will accurately translate exactly what you and the patients say. Do not speak about patients in the third person.
- Allow extra time for the interview. (Jarvis, 2000)
- Interpreters of the same gender as the patient are usually preferred.
- Do not use family members or friends as interpreters.
- Do not use minor children to interpret for LEP adults.
- Recognize the influence of religion in developing beliefs, values, and healing practices.
- Develop insight into your own attitudes, beliefs, and values.
- Avoid using your own values to judge others.
- Respect the patient's beliefs and values.
- Develop understanding of the role of the nuclear and extended families.
- Develop knowledge of cultural health beliefs, practices, and healers.
- Recognize that folk healing or traditional medicine may be practiced along with Western medicine.
- Avoid cultural stereotypes.

Adapted from *National Standards for Culturally and Linguistically Appropriate Services in Health Care*. Prepared under contract No. 282-99-0039. Rockville, MD: IQ Solutions, March 2001.

REMEMBER

Generalizations should not be applied to all members of a specific cultural or ethnic group. Communication with each patient should be individualized.

Concepts that Vary by Culture and Ethnicity*

TOUCH

- Conveys various meanings.
- Same-gender health-care provider may be preferred.
- Parental permission may be needed to touch a child.

EYE CONTACT

- Varies greatly among cultures (e.g., looking at the floor, downcast eyes).
- Conveys different meanings.

SPACE

- Value placed on space differs (e.g., territoriality).
- Size of one's intimate zone varies.
- Entry into intimate or personal space needs explanation.

TIME

- Values about past, present, and future vary.
- Values on promptness vary (e.g., following a time schedule).

SILENCE

- Uncomfortable for some.
- May convey understanding, respect, or agreement.

*Source: Adapted from Jarvis, C (ed): Physical Examination. Saunders, Philadelphis, 2000; and Kozier, B, Erb, G, Berman, A, & Snyder, SJ (eds): Fundamentals of Nursing, ed. 7. Pearson Prentice Hall, Upper Saddle River, NJ, 2004.

FORMALITY/INFORMALITY

- Varies from expectations of an authoritarian approach of the health-care professional to a close, personal relationship.

INFORMATION SHARING

- People from some cultures wait to be asked about information rather than volunteer information.

CHAPTER

Health History Guidelines

(See App. C for a sample health history form.)

Introduction

Taking the patient's health history serves a variety of purposes. First, the health history provides the patient's perspective of the database and the context of beliefs and values in which the patient operates. It communicates not only the patient's words but also the patient's nonverbal language and inflections of voice. Second, taking the health history offers an opportunity to establish rapport with the patient. The interviewer can demonstrate interest in the patient and the health condition and can encourage trust through both verbal and nonverbal behaviors. Third, the health history provides essential direction for the remainder of the examination. For example, the patient may describe a pattern of chronic alcohol abuse, which should guide the examiner in examining the liver and skin and indicate specific laboratory tests to pursue.

The patient is the most important source of data for both the health history and the physical examination. Sufficient time should be allowed so that the patient does not feel rushed and so that vital clues are not overlooked. Interviewing skills are improved with practice, and most nurses develop an interaction style with which they are comfortable. The nurse may occasionally need to review principles of therapeutic communication to enhance these skills.

In the case of a child or of an older patient with a family member present, taking the health history is an important time to include the family's data. The nurse can indicate the importance of the patient as the center of the nursing process, while acknowledging the value of the family's contribution. This may also be an opportunity to observe and/or explore such family problems as caregiver stress, inadequate parenting skills, insufficient social support, or even physical or psychological abuse.

Tips for Interviewing

- Sit facing the patient, if possible, so that the patient can see your face. Sitting suggests relaxation and indicates that time will be allowed for the interview.
- Provide privacy, and attend to patient comfort; for example, supply pillows for support, a footstool, or a glass of water.
- Use plain English. Avoid scientific and professional jargon and acronyms. Avoid condescension and patronizing tones.
- Explain the purpose of the interview, how long it will last, and how the information will be used.
- Take brief notes. Avoid emphasizing the notes but capture important statements accurately.
- Use open-ended questions; such as "How do the headaches begin?" to explore feelings and perceptions and to identify areas requiring follow-up.
- Use narrow questions to help the patient focus, such as "Do you have vomiting with the nausea?"
- Follow up critical areas during the initial interview. For example, a patient explains that he takes digoxin and has had nausea and vomiting for 3 days. Also, record those areas that need further exploration at a later date. For example, an adolescent patient reports that her grandmother has osteoporosis and uterine cancer.
- Look and listen carefully for clues, both verbal and nonverbal, unless contraindicated by the patient's cultural background. Establish eye contact, avoid answering for the patient, and explore clues in a nonthreatening manner.

- Avoid interruptions and the appearance of being distracted or bored, such as looking at the clock or flipping pages in the record. Wait for answers. Silence encourages thinking and often produces verbal responses.
- Avoid tiring the patient. A thorough health history may take from 20 minutes to 1 hour, the length varying according to the patient's condition and the setting.
- Use visual models to illustrate questions as appropriate.

Interviewing*

Purpose of an Interview

- To establish rapport.
- To establish or maintain nurse-patient relationship.
- To obtain information.
- To identify or clarify problems.
- To give information to the patient or to teach him or her.
- To counsel and/or assist the patient in finding solutions to problems.

Structure of the Interview

- *Directive:* One that is highly structured, through which specific information is sought
- *Nondirective:* One in which interviewer clarifies statements and encourages elaboration to assist patient in reaching conclusions

Guidelines for an Effective Interview

- Use therapeutic communication.
- Identify the needed information before the interview.
- Minimize distractions in the environment.
- Use vocabulary understandable to the patient.

*From Partnership for Clear Health Communication. (n.d.) *What Can Providers Do?* Ask Me 3. Retrieved 17 March 2004 from *http://www.askme3.org/*

- Be tactful about asking questions of a personal nature. Ask yourself. "Is this information really necessary?" If necessary, explain to patient why the information is needed.
- Be an active listener. (See guidelines for being an active and effective listener on page 7.)
- Remain alert for answers that may be socially acceptable but not entirely accurate or for answers the patient thinks the nurse wants to hear.
- Avoid rushing the patient; allow time for thought. (This is especially important in cultures where periods of silence are valued.)
- Avoid letting personal beliefs, biases, or values interfere.
- Conduct interview at eye level with patient.
- Look and listen for cues (e.g., changes in facial expression or posture) for follow-up questions.
- Ask nonleading, open-ended questions.
- Use an amplifying device (e.g., have the patient put the ear pieces of a stethoscope in his or her ears while you speak into the diaphragm, or use other assistive device) for persons with decreased hearing function.
- Avoid following a form too closely and taking extensive notes during the interview.
- Document information clearly and succinctly as soon as possible after leaving the room.
- Use direct quotes of the patient when they are especially meaningful.
- Complete the interview in less than 20 minutes if you are in an acute care setting.
- Ask patients to repeat back teaching content you cover during the interview or health history.
- At the end ask, "Is there anything else you would like to tell me?"

REMEMBER

- Summarize the interview for the patient to be sure the information is correct.
- Practice interviewing to develop your skills.

Information Needed for a Complete Health History

The assessment begins with the complete health history. This phase helps develop rapport with the patient so that he or she will feel more comfortable during the rest of the assessment. It also alerts the health-care provider about which systems and symptoms need to be assessed carefully later in the assessment process. Statements may be used, such as "I am going to be asking you some questions about your past health history so we can better determine your current needs and care." All of the previously discussed content related to communication skills and interviewing techniques are especially important during this phase of the assessment. Most health-care institutions and agencies have their own health history forms on which to record these data. A list of important information to obtain follows.

Date of Health History Personal Data

- Name
- Gender
- Date of birth
- Place of birth
- Age
- Ethnic background
- Native language
- Marital status
- Address
- Telephone number
- Name and telephone number of primary care physician (specialists, if needed)
- Hospital preferred
- Social Security number
- Medicare and/or Medicaid number
- Other insurance name and number
- Religious preference, including church, synagogue mosque, temple or other faith group membership.
- Person to be contacted in an emergency (name, relationship, address, and telephone number)

- Education (formal and informal)
- Occupation (now or before retirement)

Reason for Seeking Health Care (Chief Complaint [CC]) History of Present Illness (PI)

- Onset
- Location of symptoms
- Chronology
- Setting
- Precipitating factors
- Alleviating factors
- Aggravating factors
- Associated symptoms
- Treatments
- Patient's view of cause

Past Health History

- Patient's perception of level of health, in general
- Childhood illnesses (dates and types)
- Genogram (family history of diseases)
- Immunizations (see App. H)
- Allergies
- Serious accidents and/or injuries (types and dates)
- Major adult illnesses (types and dates)
- Behavioral problems
- Surgical procedures (types and dates)
- Other hospitalizations (types and dates)
- Obstetric history
- Date of menopause
- Environmental hazards:
  - Home
  - Work
  - Community
- Blood transfusions (given or received, dates)

Current Medications

- Ask patient to list all prescription medications he or she is taking.
- Ask patient to explain why he or she is taking each of these medications.
- Ask patient if he or she is having any difficulties in purchasing medications.
- Ask patient to list the over-the-counter (OTC) preparations he or she is taking. The use of alternative and complementary substances (e.g., herbs and large doses of multiple vitamins) is greatly increasing. Some interact with prescription medications and cause serious side and/or adverse effects. Record the names and doses of all such substances currently being taken.
- Ask patient about home remedies he or she is using.
- Ask patient if he or she is taking any borrowed medications.
- Ask patient if he or she is experiencing any side and/or adverse effects from any of the medications he or she is taking. Explain the difference between side and adverse effects.
- Assess discrepancies between prescribed frequency and dose and actual pattern of intake.
- Ask to see all medications being taken. Have the patient bring his or her medications to clinic, or check medications during each home visit.
- Instruct patient to discard discontinued or expired medication in a plastic bag in the trash.
- Instruct patient to use a medication organizer, which can be bought at a pharmacy. For home health patients, check the organizer each visit and fill p.r.n.
- Provide a Medication Card (see App. X) and help the patient complete it so that the needed information will always be available when seeking medical care.

Personal Habits and Patterns of Living

- *Work:* Type, length of time employed, stressors
- *Rest and/or sleep:* How much, when, sleep inducers
- *Physical activity:* How much, when, assistive devices
- *Recreation, leisure, hobbies:* Type, amount

- *Nutrition:* Time, foods, fluids, and amounts for all meals and snacks (24-hour recall); recent changes in appetite; special diet
- *Caffeine:* Source, amount, problems caused by caffeine
- *Alcohol and/or other drugs:* Type, number of years used, amount, perceived problems with level of use
- *Tobacco:* Type, number of years used, amount per day
- *Urinary and bowel activity:* Frequency, amount, problems
- *Sexual activity:* Level of activity, use of contraceptives, problems, sexual orientation

ACTIVITIES OF DAILY LIVING (ADL)

Ask about the patient's ability to perform (alone or with help) the following activities:

- Ambulating
- Dressing
- Grooming
- Bathing
- Toileting
- Eating
- Using the telephone
- Doing laundry
- Housekeeping
- Obtaining access to the community
- Driving
- Purchasing food
- Preparing food (See also functional assessment on page 29)
- Reading, using numbers, and using reading and numbers to manage health (health literacy)
- Using the Internet and computer

Psychosocial History

The psychosocial history is important in any assessment that considers a holistic view of the patient, especially in a community or long-term care setting. The psychosocial history involves the patient's relationship to others, such as family members, friends, neighbors, church groups, colleagues at work, and friends in social and civic organizations in the community. Assessing factual data about the patient's social network and needs is essential, but determining feelings about those contacts and needs is also important. Expression of feelings is more difficult for some patients than others, but the skillful nurse who communicates well will more likely set an environment where important feelings will be expressed.

Inquire about and document the following:

- Significant others, relationship, proximity
- Support systems needed and available:
  - *Informal:* Family, friends, neighbors
  - *Formal:* Temporary Aid to Needy Families (TANF); Medicaid: Medicare: Special Supplementary Food Program for Women, Infants, and Children (WIC): Food Stamps: Supplemental Security Income (SSI)
  - *Semiformal:* School, church, clubs
- Satisfaction with social contacts
- Typical 24-hour weekday and weekend day:
  - Satisfaction with employment
  - Recreational activities enjoyed
  - Leisure time activities pursued
  - Sports enjoyed as a participant or observer
- Living arrangements:
  - Alone, with family members, or with others
  - Number of rooms
  - Number and ages of other individuals in home
  - Feelings about home arrangements
- Significant stressors
- Coping ability
- *Feelings about self:* Self-concept, functional status, adaptations, independence, body image, marital status, sexuality, sexual orientation
- *History of interpersonal trauma:* Rape, incest, abuse as child or spouse, other personal tragedies. Note ability to discuss, current stage in resolution (denial, fear, anger, adaptation), and resources.
- Periods of grief and current status

- Understanding of and feelings about current illness(es)
- Feelings about retirement (past, present, or future)
- Psychological problems and conflicts
- Feelings about past, present, or future caregiver roles (care for children, disabled adults, older family members)
- Spiritual concerns and needs:
  - Concept of God
  - Source of strength
  - Value placed on religious practices and rituals
  - Perceived relationship between religious beliefs and patient's current state of health
  - Spiritual adviser
  - Role and relationship with an organized religious group

Mental Status Assessment

Children and Adolescents

Specific components of the mental status assessment are appropriate for most patients beginning at about age 2. Assessment of the child will include interviews with the parents about the child as well as with the child, developmental assessment, and the physical and neurologic assessments. Direct observation of the child in a familiar environment, often during play, is also important.

Adults

Mental status assessment is often neglected in the process of health assessment, especially in an acute care setting when physical signs and symptoms predominate. However, it should not be neglected because many mental health problems go undetected and eventually cause severe consequences for patients and their families. A baseline mental status assessment should be made on admission to a hospital or long-term-care facility. Patients who are acutely ill often manifest changes in mental status. For example, an older patient hospitalized for major surgery or other illness may be confused or disoriented because of *delirium* (a temporary, usually reversible, condition caused by a physical factor such as medication), but the health-care provider may assume the confusion is caused by *dementia* associated with aging (an example of ageism or myth about the aging process). Memory loss may be a symptom of depression rather than dementia. The nurse should assess, record, and report *any* changes in mental or cognitive status so that a specific diagnosis can be made and treatment started.

Assessing orientation to person, place, and time (often the *only* portion of the mental status examination made) may not be accurate or helpful in some situations. Knowledge of exact place or time may not be possible or important to some residents of long-term-care facilities because they do not have access to clocks, calendars, or daily newspapers. Some patients may be able to state person, place, and time correctly but be unable to write an organized sentence or copy a simple diagram. Therefore, a more thorough assessment should be made.

General Components of the Mental Status Assessment

- Level of consciousness
- *Appearance:* Dress, hygiene, grooming, mannerisms, gestures
- Eye contact
- Position, posture, gait
- Orientation:
  - *Person:* First and last name
  - *Place:* Name of facility or home address
  - *Time:* Year, month, date of month, day of week, season, a.m. or p.m.
- *Speech:* Volume, clarity, speed, quantity, tone, accent
- *Language:* Fluency, comprehension, word choice, native language
- *Affect:* Alert, calm, responsive
- *Mood:* Feelings such as sad, depressed, joyful
- *Memory:* Immediate, recent, remote, old
- *Intelligence:* Mental development, thinking skills, vocabulary, calculation
- *Abstract thinking:* Judgment, analogies

- *Attention span:* Intense, distracted, severely limited
- *Thought content:* Depression, paranoid beliefs, obsessions, hallucinations, phobias, delusions, illusions
- *Thought process:* Logical, spontaneous, flight of ideas, bizarre, digressive
- *Writing:* Ability to write a sentence or copy a figure
- *Insight:* Awareness and meaning of illness
- *Attitude:* Cooperative, evasive, passive, hostile
- *Activity level:* Appropriate, restless, lethargic
- *Response to assessment:* Cooperative, quiet, argumentative

Note

See the Sample Mental Status Assessment Flow Sheet (Hogstel, 1991) in App. D and the Folstein Mini-Mental State Examination (Folstein, Folstein, and McHugh, 1975) in App. E.

■ Functional Assessment

Functional assessment is an essential component of the total health assessment. Some questions to be answered include:

- Is the person functioning at the appropriate developmental level based on age and other characteristics?
- If not, exactly which functions are not being performed? What are the reasons for the lack of or difficulty in functioning?
- What is the individual patient's, family's, and health-care provider's perception or report of level of functioning? Sometimes patients report a *higher* level of functioning than do either family members or nurses. Older people particularly may rate their health as good when their health is poor based on objective data.
- What is the degree or level of functioning for each ability?
  - Completely independent (needs no assistance)
  - Minimal assistance needed to perform

- Maximum assistance needed to perform
- Completely dependent (needs total assistance)
- What assistance does the patient need to be able to function as normally as possible in society? (e.g., some patients need wheelchairs for mobility although they live alone and function well.)
- Where should the patient and family be referred to obtain the necessary assistance to maximize the patient's potential despite disabilities that limit functioning?

Functions to be Assessed (Adults)

PHYSICAL ACTIVITIES OF DAILY LIVING (PADL)

- Eating
- Bathing
- Dressing
- Grooming
- Toileting
- Transferring
- Walking

Instrumental Activities of Daily Living (IADL)

- Housekeeping
- Using the telephone
- Managing money
- Preparing meals
- Driving
- Shopping
- Traveling
- Taking medications correctly
- Taking out the garbage

It is difficult to assess the level of many of these functions in an acute care or clinical setting, especially at a time when the person is least likely to be functioning at a normal level because of the effects of an acute medical condition, surgery, anesthesia, and medications. Therefore, reports of the patient and family may be used. Observation of the performance IADLs will probably be more accurate than reports by patients or family members. Home-health-care nurses and nurses in other community settings are more likely to make accurate assessments of ongoing functional status. It is especially important for nurses to obtain an initial assessment of functional status on admission to home-health-care services, community clinics, and long-term care facilities so that status over time can be evaluated.

Functional Assessment Tests

There are numerous functional assessment tests that have been developed and used extensively.

NEWBORNS

* *Apgar Scoring System* (see App. G): This is a functional assessment test administered to newborns to assess physiologic adaptation in the first minutes of life.

INFANTS AND CHILDREN

* *Denver II Test.* This screening tool evaluates functional status in the areas of personal-social, language, fine motor, and gross motor skills in children up to age 6.

ADULTS

* *Katz Index of Independence in Activities of Daily Living* (see App. F): This is a widely used scale that assesses bathing, dressing, toileting, transfers, continence, and feeding on three levels: independent, assisted, and dependent (Katz, Ford, and Moskowitz, 1963).
* *Barthel Index.* This scale helps determine whether people are able to care for themselves and has been used to document improvement (Mahoney and Barthel, 1965).

Many health-care institutions and organizations have developed their own functional assessment tools and, in fact, qualification for covered health services (e.g., home-health-care under Medicaid) may depend on level of functional status in some states.

📖 Review of Systems (Symptoms)

The review of systems (sometimes called the *review of symptoms*) helps the nurse to focus on each major system of the body, noting from the health history which systems may have special problems. This systematic process prevents the omission of important assessment information.

See Part 3, "Body Organ and System Assessment," for specific questions to ask about each system.

- General
- Integument (skin, hair, nails)
- Head
- Eyes
- Ears
- Nose and sinuses
- Mouth and throat
- Neck
- Lungs and thorax
- Breasts and axillae
- Cardiovascular system
- Abdomen
- Musculoskeletal system
- Male genitourinary system and rectum
- Female genitourinary system and rectum
- Neurologic
- Adaptations in pregnancy

📖 Pediatric Additions to the Health History

Personal Data

- Child's nickname
- Parents' telephone numbers (home and work)
- Legal agreements affecting custody

Reason for Seeking Health Care (Chief Complaint)

- Person who wanted the child to see a health-care provider (child, parent, teacher)

History of Previous Illness

- Parents' reaction to child's illness
- Child's response to previous treatment or hospitalization

Past Health History

Mother's Health During Pregnancy

- Age
- *Any drugs taken:* Prescription, nonprescription, alcohol, illegal drugs
- Whether pregnancy was planned
- Complications
- Illnesses
- Concerns
- *Exposure to toxins or other hazards:* Radon, chemicals

Natal and Childhood History

- Length of gestation
- Location of birth
- *Type of labor:* Induced, spontaneous: less than 12 hours, greater than 24 hours
- *Delivery:* Spontaneous, forceps, cesarean section; anesthesia
- *Apgar Scoring System:* See Appendix G.
- Birth weight
- Complications

NEONATAL HISTORY

- Congenital anomalies
- Condition of infant
- Oxygen and/or ventilator use
- Estimation of gestational age
- *Problems:* Feeding, jaundice, respiratory distress
- Age at discharge from hospital
- Weight at discharge from hospital
- *First month of life:* Family adaptations, responses to baby, perceived ability of family to care for baby

INFANT AND CHILDHOOD HISTORY

- *Illnesses:* Note exposure, specific disorders, residual effects.
- *Allergies:* Note eczema, allergic rhinitis, urticaria, vomiting after introduction of new foods, diarrhea.
- *Immunizations:* Note each vaccine, age received, reactions. (See App. H for immunization schedule.)
- *Screening tests:* Note types and the child's age when each test was performed (vision, hearing, scoliosis, sickle cell disease, tuberculosis, lead).
- *Surgeries and/or hospitalizations:* Note the child's and parents' reactions to the events.
- *Accident and/or trauma history:* Note consistency of explanations and emotional response to questioning if abuse is suspected.

FEEDING HISTORY

- *Feedings and/or supplements:* Type, amount
- Weight gain
- Age at which solid foods were started
- Type of solid foods fed
- Infant's responses to foods
- Parents' responses to feeding their infant
- Weaning
- Food preferences
- *Current feeding:* Type, schedules
- Ability to feed self

DEVELOPMENTAL HISTORY (SEE ALSO APP. I FOR EXAMPLES OF PEDIATRIC DEVELOPMENTAL MILESTONES)

Note the child's height and weight at different ages, as well as the age when the child was able to do the following activities:

- Hold head up
- Roll over
- Reach for toys
- Sit alone
- Crawl
- Stand alone
- Walk
- Say first word
- Speak in two-word sentences
- Dress self
- Use the toilet (urination, defecation)

Sexual Development, Education, and Activity

- Present status of sexual development
- Age of voice change and pubic hair growth (boys)
- Age of breast development and menarche (girls)
- Social relations with same and opposite gender
- Curiosity about sexuality
- Masturbation
- Contraception
- Parental responses and instructions to the child about sexuality and dating
- Child's use of language to discuss sexuality (Note age appropriateness and indicators of precocity. Note behaviors suggestive of sexual abuse.)

Social History

- *Sleep:* Patterns, problems, terrors
- *Speech:* Stuttering, delays
- *Habits:* Rocking, nail biting
- *Discipline used:* Type, frequency, effectiveness, attitudes, response of parents to temper tantrums
- *School:* Current grade, any preschool attendance, adjustments, failures, favorite subjects, performance, problems

- *Social behavior:* Relationships with peers, parents, authority figures: type of peer group, level of independence: interests and/or hobbies: self-image (If infant, toddler, or preschooler, note child-parent interactions, demonstration of affection, willingness of child to separate from parent [least likely, age 8 to 20 months], evidence of increasing independence and competence.)

Family History

- Maternal gestational history
- Any consanguinity in family
- Employment history
- Child care arrangements
- Adequacy of clothing, food, transportation, sleep arrangements
- Parents' relationship with each other
- Parents' illnesses
- Siblings' relationship to one another
- Siblings' illnesses

Safety History
Infants and Small Children

- Use of infant seat or seat belts
- Accessibility and inaccessibility to child of poisons, household cleaning products, medications, firearms, and matches
- Presence and placement of fire extinguishers and smoke detectors
- Infants sleeping on their back or side, not abdomen
- Bottle propping
- Milk or sweetened fluids at night in crib
- Stairway gates, window guards, pool gates
- Poison control center telephone number
- Effect of passive smoking
- Temperature setting of hot water heater (should be 120°F or less [49°C or less])
- Use of bicycle helmet

Teens

- Assess tobacco, alcohol, and drug use.

- Assess sexual practices, risk of hepatitis B, human immunodeficiency virus (HIV) or other sexually transmitted diseases (STDs).
- Assess water safety practices. Remind not to swim alone or dive into water of unknown depth.

Geriatric Additions to the Health History

Immunizations

- *Pneumococcal vaccine:* Dates. If received before 1983, before age 65, or if person is at high risk of getting the disease and was immunized more than 5 years ago, revaccination may be necessary.
- *Influenza vaccine:* Date of last immunization. Recommended to be given annually from mid-October through mid-November.
- *Tetanus:* Date of last administration. Recommended every 10 years. If the individual never received a primary series against tetanus and diphtheria as a child, the adult should receive a series of three vaccinations (the first doses at least 4 weeks apart and the third dose 6 to 12 months later).

Current Prescription Medications

It is important to have the patients bring in all medications.

- Names of the medications
- Prescribing health-care professional(s)
- Prescribed dosages (assess whether the patient is overdosing or underdosing)
- Side effects and/or adverse effects
- Adherence problems
- Ability to afford the medications
- Ability to get to the pharmacy
- Difficulty swallowing
- Patient's opinion of efficacy of medications
- Patient's use of borrowed medications
- Understanding of total medication regimen (purpose,

method, timing, action, dose, side effects, adverse effects, interactions)
- Use of any memory aids (e.g., pill boxes, alarm)
- Difficulty administering the medications (visual impairments, cognitive impairments, problems with manual dexterity)

Current over-the-counter (OTC) Medications

- Names of the medications
- *Dosages:* Amount, frequency (especially note high doses of vitamins)
- Reasons for taking medications
- Side effects or adverse effects
- Home remedies, folk medicine, herbal preparations

Nutrition

- *Salt and sugar intake:* Note whether the patient adds salt or sugar to food at the table or in cooking: the amount of sugar used on cereal and in coffee and/or tea: other food items with high salt or sugar content.
- *Weight:* Note any weight changes (increase or decrease) in the patient over the past month, year, or 5 years. Patient's perception of weight.
- *Special diet:* If the patient is on a special diet, note the type and any difficulty following the diet. Assess knowledge of diet. Does the patient use any dietary supplements (kind, amount, frequency)?
- *Food preferences:* Note patient's current food likes or dislikes, amounts of food consumed at one time, frequency of meals, typical meals.
- *Appetite:* Note whether the patient's hunger is more pronounced at certain times of the day or night; any loss of or increase in appetite recently or over the past year; any recent changes in kinds of food eaten.
- *Food purchase and preparation:* Note who buys and prepares the food and whether the patient likes it. If patient prepares his or her own food, note whether preparation is a problem. If so,

is problem caused by fatigue, eating alone, decreased vision, memory impairment, or difficulty using any appliances?

- *Ingestion:* Note any difficulty the patient has in feeding self, chewing, swallowing, or choking. Are there any tooth or mouth problems? Does the patient have dentures and, if so, are they in good repair, do they fit properly, and does the patient wear them? Are there certain consistencies of food the patient avoids?

- *Affordability:* Note whether the patient is able to afford the food needed and desired.

Activities of Daily Living (ADL) (See also App. F)

Note whether the patient requires any assistance in the following ADLs:

- *Dressing:* Fastening buttons, zippers; tying shoes
- *Grooming and hygiene:* Trimming fingernails or toenails, shaving, brushing teeth, brushing hair
- *Bathing:* Preparing bathwater, for tub or shower, getting into or out of the tub or shower, washing all body parts
- *Toileting:* Continence—getting into the bathroom, getting onto and/or off the commode, hygiene after elimination
- *Mobility:* Getting into and/or out of bed, lowering into and/or getting up from chairs, transferring from bed to chair, walking, climbing stairs, reaching for items in cupboards, opening doors, recent falls
- *Eating:* Handling utensils, cutting food, putting food into mouth
- *Laundry:* Washing by hand or using washing machine
- *Meal preparation:* Planning, preparing, and serving adequate meals
- *Housekeeping:* Making the bed, cleaning the house, washing the dishes, taking out the garbage
- *Financial affairs:* Paying bills, balancing the checkbook
- *Shopping:* Transporting to store, making selections, paying for items appropriately

- *Medication administration:* Complying with regimen, medication set up, or assistance needed
- *Transportation:* Public transit, drives own car, relies on friends and/or family, public agency

> **Note**
>
> If the patient needs assistance with any of the previous ADLs, determine the amount of assistance needed and any adaptive equipment used. Does the patient have adequate support systems available to provide the necessary assistance needed? Do family and/or friends know where and how to access the needed services?

Social Support and/or Resources (See also App. J)

- *Community involvement:* Faith group involvement, volunteer work, employment, hobbies, group memberships, social and/or recreational programs, classes
- *Support system:* Family and/or friends, amount of contact, type of relationship and contact, pets
- *Living arrangement:* Who lives with patient and where does patient live (own home, apartment, retirement community, nursing home, assisted living facility)
- *Finances:* Amount and/or source of income, type of health insurance coverage, perception of adequacy of income to meet needs
- *Legal services:* Assistance used. Does patient have a will, a durable Power of Attorney, a Medical Power of Attorney, or other advance directive?
- *Community services:* Does the patient use such services as homemaker services, adult day services, home health care, meal assistance programs and/or nutrition sites, financial assistance programs, senior centers, home repair services, rehabilitation services?

Demographic Characteristics in the United States

    Table 3-1

A Profile of the United States, 2000

Characteristic	% of population
People less than 18 years old	25.7
People 65 years and older	12.4
People who report being Caucasian only	75.1
People who report being African-American only	12.3
People who report being Native-American and Alaskan Native only	0.9
People who report being Asian only	3.6
People who report being Native Hawaiian and other Pacific Islander only	0.1
People who report being 2 or more races	2.4
People who report being of Hispanic or Latino origin	12.5
People who were foreign born	11.1
People, aged 5 and older, who speak a language other than English at home	17.9
People, aged 5 and older, who report a disability	19.0

U.S. Census 2000.

Cultural Assessment*

National Standards for Culturally and Linguistically Appropriate Services in Health Care United States Department of Health and Human Services Office of minority Health, Washington, DC (USDHHS), office of minority Health, Washington, DC, March 2001. Call for culturally competent care. Prepared under contract No. 282-99-039. Rockville, Md, IQ Solutions. Learning to be culturally competent is a lifelong endeavor for nurses. Because health and health care are social constructs, learning to be culturally aware, culturally sensitive, and ultimately culturally competent is essential for optimal nursing care.

Culture: *Learned, integrated* patterns of thinking, believing, and behaving *shared* by people. Culture is expressed in many ways, including customs, dress, role definitions, perceptions and expectations, communication, beliefs, values, morals, dietary practice, and art. Most people are multicultural; they belong to more than one culture.

Cultural and linguistic competence: "a set of congruent behaviors, attitudes, and policies that come together in a system, agency, or among professionals that enables effective work in cross-cultural situations.... *Competence* implies having the capacity to function effectively as an individual and an organization within the context of the cultural beliefs, behaviors, and needs presented by consumers and their communities" (USDHHS, Mar 2001, p. 131).

CLIENTS HAVE THE RIGHT TO

- Health care that is compatible with their cultural beliefs, practices, and preferred language
- Health-care providers with adequate training and ongoing education in culturally and linguistically appropriate health-care delivery
- Appropriate and qualified language assistance services at no additional cost
- Easily understood patient-related materials (adapted from USDHHS, Mar 2001)

NURSES CAN DEVELOP CULTURAL COMPETENCE BY

- Becoming aware of their own cultures and how those cultures influence practice.
- Getting to know patients as individuals and families. People are unique and rarely match a cultural profile or stereotype.
- Participating in ongoing formal and informal educational opportunities, including community events and celebrations related to various cultures.
- Avoiding ethnocentric behavior—the belief that their cultural beliefs and behaviors are superior to other cultural beliefs and behaviors.

SELECTED CULTURAL TRAITS OF PATIENTS

PHYSICAL APPEARANCE

- Hairstyle and ornamentation
- Posture, facial expressions, body language

- Grooming and personal hygiene
- Dress

Mental Characteristics and Psychological Orientation (Mind)

- Self-identification of race, ethnicity, and other cultures
- Emotional disposition, temperament
- Sensory acuity: Visual, auditory, tactile, olfactory
- Personal traits
- Mental health status

Social and Physical Environments

- Ancestry, geographic origin
- Current geographic location, geographic and climatic features
- Organization of and strength of family unit
- Languages and communication patterns
- Expectations and behavioral norms for age, gender, and role
- Format (rituals) for major life events: Birth, puberty, marriage, illness, death
- Economic and work opportunities and access to resources
- Housing and living arrangements
- Dominant and minority faith practices
- Beliefs about disease causation
- Availability, quality, and variety of health-care services
- Political and governmental structure
- Dietary customs, access to adequate amounts and quality of food
- Community resources for education, art, music, recreation

Internal Synthesis of Body, Mind, and Environment (Self)

- Self-concept, self-perception, expectations of self
- Beliefs, values, spirituality, religious affiliation
- Affect, mood, congruity between words and affect
- *Personal goals—:* Short-term and long-term
- *Work role:* Economic contribution to self others
- Areas of accomplishment, achievement; sources of pride

- Knowledge base, use of educational opportunities
- Response to stress, coping strategies, ability to adapt
- *Language usage:* Formal, slang, dialect
- Food preferences, dietary restrictions
- Interests in applied and fine arts, crafts, hobbies, music, literature
- Reading ability and preference
- Use of technology, computer, Internet

Cultural Assessment Guide

The cultural nursing assessment is the systematic appraisal of individuals or groups about cultural beliefs, values, and practices to determine nursing needs and interventions based on cultural factors. The cultural nursing assessment provides an extended data collection tool for the recording of pertinent cultural factors that are vital to the patient's acceptance of and adherence to the medical regimen, nursing interventions, and behavior modification plans. The cultural aspects of the patient's lifestyle, health beliefs, and health practices are essential elements that will enhance the nurse's decision making and judgment when planning and providing effective nursing care.

A thorough cultural assessment should be implemented during the initial history-taking interview with each patient. The cultural assessment guide will provide documentation of the information concerning the patient's traditional cultural values and beliefs, communication and language patterns, and most importantly, the daily living patterns. The cultural assessment guide will also serve as a reference for other members of the health-care team when providing care. The nurse will analyze the data, formulate goals with the patient when necessary, implement nursing interventions, and evaluate the goals.

The nurse should be prepared to interview the patient and obtain as much information as possible concerning the patient's dominant cultural group practices. The nurse plans for an organized sequence of data collection with specific assessment categories in which information about the patient is gathered. The major categories of a comprehensive cultural assessment should include the following items:

- Historical origin of the cultural group:
  - History and origin of ancestors
  - Length of time in original country and in current environment
- Physical presentation:
  - Attire, demeanor, relationship of person(s) accompanying the patient
- Communication and language patterns:
  - Literacy
  - Dominant language used in the home and understanding of the English language
  - Verbal and nonverbal messages and meanings
  - Titles, proper forms of greetings, and respect
  - Improper topics of conversation
- Values and belief systems:
  - Worldview
  - Traditional values and adaptations to dominant culture norms
  - Code of conduct (ethics), behavior patterns, authority, responsibility
  - Attitudes toward time, work, play, money, education
- Religious beliefs, practices, and rituals:
  - *Type:* Traditional or modern
  - Symbols of worship, important emblems, icons
  - *Rituals and/or traditions:* Special celebrations, holidays (fertility, birth, puberty, marriage, death)
- Family roles and relationships:
  - Relative patterns
  - Marriage
  - *Family functions:* Organizations, roles, activities
  - Parenting styles
- Support systems:
  - Extended family organization and members.
  - Community resources
  - Cultural group affiliations

- Social systems:
  - Economics
  - Political
  - Education
- Diet, food habits, and rituals:
  - Beliefs and significance of food
  - Adaptations when cultural food is not available
  - Rituals
- Health and illness belief systems
  - Values and beliefs
  - Use of nontraditional, folklore remedies, and treatments
  - Acceptance and use of traditional and alternative health-care services
  - Health and/or illness behaviors and decision making

The nurse should communicate directly with the patient when the individual's health condition permits. However, there are very likely to be other significant people in the patient's life with whom the nurse will be required to interact when completing the cultural nursing assessment. When caring for patients from culturally diverse backgrounds, it is necessary to identify those significant others whom the patient perceives to be important and who may be responsible for decision making that affects his or her health care. The nurse should be informed about the cultural values and traditions when working with a specific cultural group and enhance these cultural norms whenever possible. Consequently, supportive family members and significant others are very important factors in patients' decision making and should be included as active participants during the cultural nursing assessment.

It is also very important for the nurse to consider that during the cultural nursing assessment, all historic reminiscences will not be pleasant for the culturally diverse patient. Consequently, recalling memories of traditional values, beliefs, rituals, former homelands, and family members can evoke very strong emotions for the patient. The nurse should be prepared to provide the culturally appropriate support to the patient. The nurse should be respectful, empathetic, supportive, facilitating, and understanding. A quiet environment that allows enough time for the patient to provide the information should be maintained, and, above all, effective listening skills should be used by the nurse.

Learner Assessment

- Prior learning experience and experiences with change.
- Learning style. There are many tools to assess learning style and several frameworks for analyzing learning style. At a minimum, try to determine the strength of patients' preferences for learning new things by reading about and looking at them, hearing about them, or doing something with them.
- Assess numeracy, the ability to use numbers for daily activities as well as literacy.
- Motivational strategies that help patients learn.
- Readiness to learn or make changes.

Family Assessment*

- Interview all family members at the same time to observe communication and decision-making patterns.
- Families take many forms: Nuclear conjugal families, extended families, single-parent families, stepfamilies, cohabiting families, gay and lesbian families, and communal families.
- Collect and analyze information about the whole family and its individual members related to:
  - Biological and physiologic function
  - Psychologic function, particularly
    - Communication patterns
    - Power and leadership in the family
    - Emotional strengths and coping strategies
    - Beliefs about child rearing and discipline
    - Family goals
  - Physical living environment
    - Home
    - Neighborhood and larger community

*United States Department of Health and Human Services, Office of Minority Health: National Standards for Culturally and Linguistically Appropriate Services in Health Care, Final Report. March, 2001, Contract No. 282-99-0039. Washington, D.C.: IQ Solutions.

- Sociocultural considerations
  - Formal and informal roles
  - Faith practices
  - Socioeconomic status, adequacy of financial resources
  - Employment or occupational factors
  - External social resources
- Collective family and individual member behaviors, such as:
  - Consumption of goods, services, money, information
  - Use of leisure time and participation in physical activity
  - Safety practices inside and outside the home
- Collective family and individual member
  - Responses to health and illness
  - Interactions with and use of formal and informal health systems
  - Health promotion and prevention beliefs and actions
- Assess family developmental stage:
  - Leaving home, single young adults; responsibility for self
  - New couple; commitment to a new family
  - Families with young children; accepting new family members
  - Families with adolescents; increasing flexibility to respond to adolescents' independence and elders' changing independence
  - Launching children and moving on; accepting many exits and entries into family
  - Families in later life; accepting new and shifting generational roles
  - Draw a genogram to visually represent family information over three or more generations
- Assess family's health history:
  - Include at least three generations back
  - Include ages at death and causes of death
  - Note patterns of illness distribution across generations (e.g., cancer and heart disease)
- *Assess family structure:* Single, nuclear, nuclear dyad, extended and/or multigenerational, single parent, stepfamily, same gender

- Draw an ecomap to visually represent relationships and their strengths inside and outside families (Clark, 2002).
- Assess family roles:
  - Formal roles:
    - Breadwinner(s)
    - Homemaker(s)
    - Child rearer(s)
    - Financial manager(s)
    - Chauffeur(s)
    - Cook(s)
    - House repairers
  - Informal roles (selected):
    - Encourager (praises others)
    - Harmonizer (mediator)
    - Blocker (opposer)
    - Compromiser (yielder, comes halfway)
    - Dominator (manipulator)
    - Blamer (faultfinder)
    - Scapegoat (recipient of family's hostilities)
    - Caregiver (nurturer)
- Assess family health:
  - Concepts of health and illness
  - Perceived level of health
  - Family health promotion strategies
  - Family stressors
  - Family strengths
  - Support systems
  - Family diet, mealtime practices, who prepares meals
  - Family activities
  - Time taken for sharing
  - Spirituality
  - Participation in the community
  - Is home a place for respite, for nurturing?
  - Health seeking behaviors:
    - Physical examinations
    - Dental care

- • Family physician
- • Emergency department use
- • Immunization status
- Source of insurance, adequacy of coverage
- Assess family income:
  - Source(s)
  - Adequacy
- Assess family power (Friedman 1992):
  - Assess who makes decisions:
    - • Household management
    - • Discipline of children
    - • Financial matters
    - • Health care
    - • Family leisure—time activities
  - Assess who makes the decision and/or wins when major decisions are made.
  - Assess type and sources of power used by family.
  - *Legitimate:* One person is the authority, and this authority is believed by all family members to be appropriate.
  - *Helpless and/or powerless:* The victims (disabled family members or the children, for instance) gain power secondary to their helplessness.
- *Referent power:* Power gained from family member's positive identification (parental power).
- *Resource and/or expert power:* Power is based on who has the most resources (attributes, possessions, expertise). For example, family member who controls the finances may control decision making, in general.
- *Reward power:* When one family member has the power to reward other members.
- *Coercive power:* When power is gained through the use of violence, threats, or coercion.
- *Informational power:* Power gained by persuasion.
- *Affective power:* When power is gained by controlling the allocation of affection or sex.

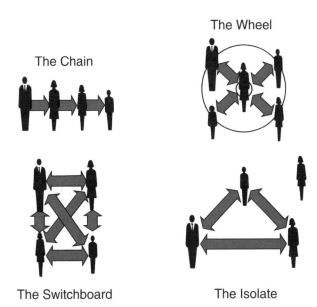

FIGURE 3-1   Family communication patterns.

- *Tension management power:* When power is gained through the use of tears, disagreements, or pouting.
- Assess power or decision-making process:
  - *Consensus:* Mutual agreement
  - *Accommodation:* Concessions made
  - *De facto:* No decisions made
- Assess family communication patterns (Fig. 3–1):
  - *Dysfunctional patterns:*
    - *The wheel:* One person directs all communication
    - *The chain:* Communication goes "down the line" without opportunity for interaction
    - *The isolate:* One person excluded
  - *Functional pattern of communication:* The switchboard (communication between all members in all directions)

- Assess family developmental stage:*
  - Beginning family: Establish marriage.
  - Early childbearing family: Stabilize family, facilitate developmental needs of family members.
  - Family with preschool children: Maintain marriage, nurture and socialize children.
  - Family with school-age children: Maintain marriage, socialize children, and promote their school achievement.
  - Family with teenagers: Maintain marriage, maintain parent-child communication, build foundation for future family stages, balance teen freedom/responsibility.
  - Launching family: Readjust marriage, launch children as young adults, assist aging parents.
  - Middle-age family: Strengthen marriage, maintain relationship with children/parents, provide healthy environment, cultivate leisure activities.
  - Aging family: Adjust to retirement, reduced income, health problems, death of spouse: maintain satisfactory living arrangement.
  - Parenting practices:
    - Hoping and planning for children
    - Uses parenting styles learned from own parents
    - Disciplines children
    - Empowers children
    - Develops positive attitudes in children toward education, religion, athletics, extracurricular activities
    - Role models for children and teaches altruism, respect for others
  - Draw ECOMAP depicting family in the center circle with spokes drawn to interacting systems. Depict direction of energy exchange and presence of stressful or tenuous relationships (see Fig. 3–2).

---

*Source: Adapted from Stanhope, M, Lancaster, J: Community Health Nursing, ed. 6. Mosby, St Louis No., 2004; and Clark, MJ: Community Health Nursing: Caring for Populations, ed. 4. Pearson Education, Upper Saddle River, NJ, 2002.

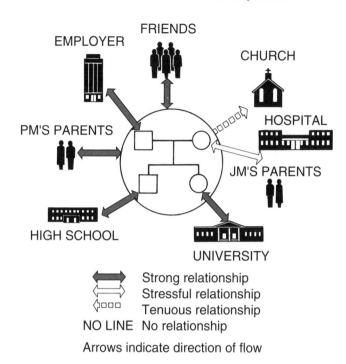

FIGURE 3-2   ECOMAP depicting family and interacting systems.

Family Caregiver Assessment

When one family member is ill or disabled, another family member often takes over the role of family caregiver. In home health or hospice settings, that role often makes the difference whether the family member can remain at home. The nurse in those settings will need to conduct either a complete family assessment or at least the following, more focused family caregiver assessment:

Overview

* Age
* Relationship to care recipient
* Number of months since onset in caregiving
* Number of hours per day spent in caregiving
* Feelings toward caregiving: Both negative and positive, advantages and disadvantages
* Knowledge of care recipient's care needs (physical and emotional)
* Knowledge of care recipient's medications
* Knowledge of what is involved in the care
* Evaluation of whether care recipient can be left alone
* Evaluation of what care recipient can do for himself or herself
* Evaluation of whether the care recipient's dependency has increased in the last month
* Personal medical problems
* Personal medications
* Personal illness patterns
* Personal sleep patterns:
  * Length
  * Pattern of interrupted or uninterrupted sleep
  * Place for caregiver to sleep
* Personal nutrition
* Personal exercise
* Personal stress reduction activities
* Frequency of leaving the home: Purpose, duration
* Availability and use of respite services: Hospital, nursing facility, family, friends, church
* Number of times in last year care recipient has been hospitalized
* Number of times in last year care recipient was hospitalized to provide caregiver with needed rest
* Assistance caregiver identifies as being needed

If the care recipient is a patient of home health care, assess if caregiver also is in need of, and potentially eligible for, home health services:

- Is the care recipient confined to the home? Confined to bed?
- Does she or he need skilled care such as direct care, teaching, or monitoring of a changing condition by a registered and/or licensed nurse?
- Is she or he under the care of a physician, who agrees that home-health-care services are needed and orders them?

Environmental Assessment

Hospital or Nursing Facility

- Observe the patient's facial expression and posture in bed.
- Note the placement and position of bed.
- Check the bed and bed rails for proper functioning and position.
- Assess any equipment attached to the patient and/or bed such as nasogastric tubing, urinary catheter, IV, or monitor for proper functioning.
- Make sure that the call cord, the telephone, paper wipes, and water (if allowed) are within easy reach of the patient.
- Note whether privacy and space for the patient's personal possessions are adequate.
- Note any unusual odors emanating from the patient or in the room.
- Note whether the floor is free from litter and moisture.
- Make sure no unnecessary equipment and/or supplies are in the room.
- Make sure lighting is adequate.

Home*

- *Neighborhood location:* Urban, suburban, rural
- Sidewalks, paved streets, presence of churches, schools, playgrounds, industries and/or businesses
- Traffic patterns in neighborhood

*Source: Adapted from Browning, M: Home environment assessment guide. In Hogstel, M (ed): Nursing Care of the Older Adult, ed. 3, Delmar, Albany, NY. 1994, pp 592–595.

- *Size and type of home:* Apartment, house, trailer
- Description of home
- Whether patient owns or rents the home
- Length of time in current home
- Distance to shopping
- Type of water supply
- Type of sewage disposal
- Type and efficiency of heating and cooling systems
- *Method of transportation:* Car, bus, walking
- Presence of a telephone or emergency signaling system
- *Neighbors:* Proximity: Whether patient perceives as supportive or threatening
- Adequacy of lighting outside and inside, including night-lights
- Distance to street lights, fire hydrant, fire station
- Visibility of path from car to house by neighbors
- General cleanliness and whether home is infested with insects or rodents
- Safety of the inside and outside stairs, number of steps
- Security of the outside doors
- *Activities of neighborhood residents:* Children at play outdoors, transient persons, older residents visibility, activity after dark
- Patient's perception of safety for self in environment; patient's awareness of crimes in area, perception of own vulnerability; degree to which precautions or fear affects daily activities
- Availability of safe source of heat and, if appropriate, air-conditioning
- Presence, placement, and functioning of smoke alarms
- Presence and placement of fire extinguishers
- Safety of the bathroom floor, tub, commode; functioning of the fixtures; raised toilet seat, grab bars near toilet and/or in tub, shower seat
- Temperature of the hot water 120°F or less (49°C or less).
- *Condition of the floors and stairs:* Cleanliness, evenness, freedom from clutter, presence of throw rugs, adequacy of lighting at night
- Width of hallways and doorways for maneuverability of walker or wheelchair

- Proximity of bathroom to bedroom
- Hospital bed located for convenience of family caregivers and for opportunity of interaction with family
- Safety and state of repair of the furniture
- Safe use of appliances and electrical cords
- Functioning refrigerator, stove
- Presence of books, radio, television, newspaper, magazines
- Computer and internet access
- Proper storage of household cleaners
- Proper storage of food and medicines
- Availability of laundry facilities
- Availability and functioning of lawn equipment

Environmental Assessment

- Potential Exposures
  - Note whether illness occurred after contact with a chemical, pesticide, or other substance.
  - Have there been symptoms that improve when away from home, work, or school?
  - At *present work* (or school):
    - Note exposure to solvents, dusts, fumes, radiation, loud noise, pesticides, or other chemicals
    - Presence of Material Data Safety Sheets on chemicals at work
    - Personal protective equipment available and required
    - Work clothes remain at work site
    - Coworkers with similar health problems
  - Past work—investigate past work (or school) experiences, length of job, military service, farm, or seasonal work
  - Residence—note when residence built, type of heating, recently remodeled chemicals stored on property, source of drinking water
  - Neighborhood—environmental concerns related to air, water, or soil; industries, farms or presence of a hazardous waste site or landfill nearby
  - Activities—activities and hobbies that engage in burning, soldering, or melting any products; participate in garden-

ing, fishing, or hunting; use game or home-grown food; use of pesticides; use of alternative healing or cultural practices

- Referrals and Resources
  - Agency for Toxic Substances and Disease Registry, www.atsdr.cdc.gov
  - Association for Occupational and Environmental Clinics, www.aoec.org
  - Environmental Protection Agency, www.epa.gov
  - Material Safety Data Sheets, www.hazard.com/msds
  - Occupational Safety and Health Administration, www.osha.gov
  - Local Health Department, Environmental Agency, Poison Control Center

▊ Summary at End of Total Health History

Ask whether there is anything else that the patient would like to tell or ask you.

Source: Adapted from Agency for Toxic Substances and Disease Registry: Environmental Exposure History, contact: www.atsdr.cdc.gov, 2001.

PART 2

The Physical Examination

CHAPTER **4**

Physical Examination Guidelines

See Appendix K for a Sample Adult Physical Assessment Form with Guide, Appendix L for the Seven Warning Signs of Cancer, and Appendix M for a Suggested Schedule of Health Screening for People Age 65 and Older with No Symptoms.

Introduction

The physical examination generally follows the history. There are several purposes for the examination. First, baseline norms are established for the patient such as skin color, temperature, heart rate, and rhythm. Second, the patient's physical status is accurately described, identifying potential and actual health problems. Third, the examination allows the nurse to document history data, such as auscultating a cardiac arrhythmia after the patient has described breathlessness and a fast pulse.

The physical examination is an important step in the establishment of a therapeutic relationship with the patient. The patient's personal needs for such things as warmth or modesty should be acknowledged and respected. The purposes of the examination are explained, and the patient should be encouraged to ask questions and give responses. This is an excellent opportunity for teaching, and the examination procedures can be practiced with accompanying teaching; for example, a heart rate of 76 is normal for the patient's age and activity.

Preparation Guidelines

- Provide a warm, comfortable, private environment with natural lighting, if possible.
- Eliminate distractions and disruptions.
- Check all needed equipment for proper functioning, and place it within easy reach. Explain equipment as it is used.
- Introduce yourself to the patient by name and title if you have not already met the patient. Unless you are in an acute care setting or an emergency department, it is preferable to meet the patient in a less threatening manner (e.g., with the patient clothed, sitting, and giving history data).
- Have the patient void before the examination; collect clean specimen, if needed.
- Explain each step as the examination progresses. Tell the patient how much time will be involved in the entire examination. Offer general health promotion guidance with each system; (e.g., explain that a breast self-examination should be performed every month).
- Avoid telling jokes, inappropriate familiarity, and casual or careless touching.
- Warm your hands and instruments before touching the patient's skin.

Physical Examination Guidelines

- If you are right-handed, stand on the patient's right side. Move to the patient's back (for posterior thorax) and to the patient's left side (for left eye), as needed. You should be able to circle the bed or table.
- Drape the patient well, exposing only those areas that are being examined.
- Be aware of your nonverbal communication during the examination; avoid frightening, intimidating, or embarrassing the patient.
- Warn the patient when any part of the examination may be uncomfortable.
- Be as gentle as possible.

- Be especially careful when examining sensitive areas (eyes, breasts, genitals).
- Always wear gloves when you may come in contact with body fluids or open lesions or if you have open areas in your skin.
- Carefully assess those areas where potential problems or concerns were discovered in the history and review of systems.
- See Appendix P for physical signs of malnutrition and deficiency state.

Techniques in Physical Assessment

Inspection

This step is observation and visual examination. It is systematic, orderly, and purposeful, for example, examining the skin for color and hair growth patterns. Inspection requires good lighting, preferably natural daylight. The area to be inspected must be fully exposed and observable. Systematically observe color, size, shape, symmetry, and position of any lesions. See Appendix K for specific examples of each of these descriptors. Inspection may include asking the patient to perform certain tasks, such as exhaling against pursed lips. Inspection may also include touch, such as squeezing the fingers and assessing blood return. Note any impairment of function.

Auscultation

This examination technique consists of listening to sounds within the body, such as the sounds of respiration or peristalsis. Most auscultation is indirect and involves the use of a stethoscope. Direct auscultation uses only the nurse's ears, and may be used to identify crepitus or an asthmatic wheeze.

The stethoscope should be no longer than 12 inches and short enough to be functional and comfortable. The flat diaphragm is used to hear higher-pitched sounds, and the bell is used to hear lower-pitched sounds:

- Use stethoscope diaphragm for bowel, breath, and cardiac sounds. Use bell for vascular and cardiac sounds.
- Assess for loudness, pitch, quality or nature, frequency, and duration (see Table 4–1).

Table 4-1

AUSCULTATION SOUNDS

Type	Description	Example
Frequency	Number of oscillations generated per second by a vibrating object	Breath and bowel sounds
Loudness	The amplitude of a sound wave	Loud or soft
Quality	The physical quality of sound	Musical or humming
Duration	Length of time sound vibrations last	Short, medium, or long

Source: Adapted from Potter, PA, & Perry, AG: Fundamentals of Nursing, ed. 5. Mosby, St Louis, MO, 2001, pp. 730–731.

Percussion (See Fig. 4–1)

In this examination technique, the examiner thumps an area of the body and observes for vibrations or sounds. Indirect percussion is the most common method, and it involves the nurse's striking a finger that is placed on the patient's body part.

Percussion requires knowledge of anatomic location of internal organs and their approximate size. The technique is a nonintrusive way of determining the size of organs and masses. It may also be used to estimate the tissue and contents of an organ or mass (e.g., a solid mass or a bladder filled with urine).

- *Indirect method:* Place middle finger only of nondominant hand on area to be percussed. Using the tip of the middle fingernail of the dominant hand, strike the nondominant resting finger with a quick bouncing blow. Compare the sounds on the right and left sides of the area being percussed, and compare the sounds with the percussion sounds chart (see Table 4–2).

Palpation

This examination technique uses touch to gather data. The fingertips are most often used to palpate lightly (e.g., to elicit inci-

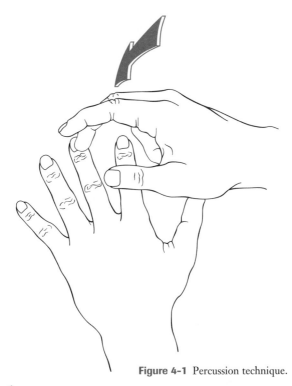

Figure 4-1 Percussion technique.

Table 4-2

PERCUSSION SOUNDS

Tone	Characteristics	Possible Source
Tympanic	Loud, clear, drumlike	Low density, such as abdominal distention with gas
Resonant	Hollow, loud	Mixed density, such as healthy lung
Hyperresonant	Echoing, hollow	Mixed density, such as emphysematous lung
Dull	Quiet, thudding	High density, such as liver
Flat	Quiet, short, flat	High density, such as bone, thick muscle

sional pain) or deeply (e.g., to determine the presence of a kidney) Deep palpation is rarely indicated in general nursing practice.

Assisting the patient to relax during palpation, especially when examining the abdominal area, will enhance the accuracy of the findings. Allow the patient to control the timing of the palpation, and be alert to cues of discomfort.

METHOD

- Palpation requires touching with different parts of the hand and with varying degrees of pressure to determine characteristics of pain, temperature, size, shape, moisture, and/or texture.
- Explain reason for touch to patient. Warm hands.
- Use light palpation before deep palpation.
- Use pads of fingers (most sensitive part) to identify texture, size, shape, or movement (e.g., pulse).
- Use dorsum of fingers for temperature assessment.
- Gently pinch skin to assess turgor on forehead or upper third of sternum.
- Use palms or ulnar side of hand to assess vibrations.
- Use deep palpation gently and briefly to assess areas, such as pelvis and abdomen for body organs and masses.
- Palpate painful areas last.

Continuing Assessment

Anytime the patient has new symptoms and/or a change in condition, an appropriate physical assessment should be performed. New symptoms, such as pain, fever, difficulty seeing, garbled speech, numbness of extremities, or sudden confusion indicate the need for a partial assessment of specific systems.

PAIN

- Assess the time of onset, site, degree, and possible contributing factors. See Figure 5–1 for a pain scale.

FEVER

- Assess all vital signs, lung sounds, urinary output.

📖 Pediatric Adaptations

General Guidelines

- If the child does not know you, it is best if there is someone else in the room whom the child trusts, preferably a parent or other family member.
- Parents can assist by telling you how they cope with the child.

Suggestions for Specific Age Groups

YOUNGER INFANTS

- Let the parent assist by holding the child on his or her lap.
- Avoid chilling the child.

OLDER INFANTS

- Parents should be within the child's view.
- Move slowly, and approach the child slowly.
- Restrain the child adequately and gently with parents' assistance.

TODDLERS AND PRESCHOOLERS

- Keep the parents in the room; ask them to assist, when appropriate.
- Tell the child that it is all right to cry or yell.
- Allow the child to play with the equipment if desired (during the history taking).
- Use distraction.
- Perform the least threatening parts of the examination first.
- Use a doll to demonstrate certain parts of the examination.
- Restrain the child adequately.
- Use the parents to assist (e.g., holding stethoscope on the child's chest).
- Give the child simple choices, when possible.

PRESCHOOLERS

- Explain briefly what the child will experience.

- Demonstrate the equipment; allow the child to play with it or use it on a doll.
- Let the child know that the examination is not punishment.
- Involve the child by allowing him or her to hold the chart or stethoscope for you.
- Praise the child for helping and cooperating.

SCHOOL-AGE CHILDREN

- Explain the examination and allow time for questions.
- Explain what you are doing.
- Allow the child to assist by handing equipment to you.
- Allow the child to listen, feel, or see what you find.
- Protect the child's privacy.

ADOLESCENTS

- Explain the examination and encourage questions.
- Examine the adolescent apart from the parents and ask if there are any questions.
- Tell the adolescent the findings and the norms (e.g., "Your breasts are beginning to develop; that is normal for a 12-year-old.").
- Protect the adolescent's privacy.

◼ Geriatric Adaptations

General Guidelines

- Prepare the environment, taking into account sensory and musculoskeletal changes:
  - Allow adequate space to accommodate mobility aids.
  - Use straight-backed chairs rather than low, soft, curved chairs.
  - Minimize background noise and distraction, such as TV, radio, intercom system, or nearby communication between other people.
  - Avoid glossy or highly polished surfaces (floors, walls, ceilings, or furnishings).

- Use a well-padded, low examination table.
- Maintain proximity to rest room facilities.
- Diffuse lighting with increased illumination (avoid using direct or fluorescent lighting). Avoid having patient face glare from windows.
- Ensure a comfortable, warm room temperature.
- Maintain complete privacy for patient.
- Conduct the examination, taking into account the energy level, pace, and adaptability of the older adult:
  - Allow ample time for the exam because older patients may move more slowly and take longer to react and respond to questions. Be alert to signs of fatigue, and consider conducting the exam in more than one session.
  - Approach the patient in a relaxed and unhurried manner.
  - Allow the patient ample time to respond to questions and directions.
  - Use silence to allow the older patient time to collect thoughts before responding.
  - Sit facing the patient to facilitate eye contact, lip reading, and rapport (see Fig. 4–2).
  - Use commonly accepted vocabulary and clear questions or instructions.
  - A visual deficit may warrant the use of frequent verbal cues and touch.
  - A hearing deficit calls for lowering the voice pitch, speaking slowly, and avoiding shouting. You may need to write information or use an amplified listening device.
  - Never leave older patients unattended on an exam table, as they could fall off while adjusting their position.
  - Assist the older patient on and off the examination table and with position changes to avoid injuries.
  - To conserve the patient's energy, organize the examination to minimize position changes.
  - To avoid chilling and protect modesty, keep the patient warmly covered and expose only the body part being examined.

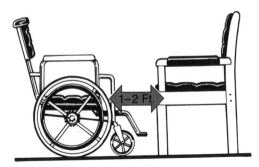

Sitting in chair or wheelchair:
  Sit very close to patient (1–2 feet away) and
  face the patient.

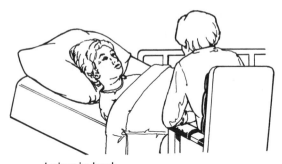

Lying in bed:
  Sit level with the patient and maintain
  a close position facing the patient.

Figure 4-2 Optimal seating positions for communication with the older adult.

Possible Modifications

• If the patient has breathing problems or a curvature of the spine, it may be necessary to elevate the examining table and/or use pillows.

- If the patient has a musculoskeletal disorder and/or feels dizzy, some neurologic tests may need to be omitted.

Cultural Considerations

- When patients are culturally different from the nurse, the physical exam may require additional time because of language differences, increased sensitivity to exposure, observation and palpation of body parts, and the proximity of the nurse to the patient.
- Be aware of nonverbal communication during the examination. Avoid sudden moves, extreme facial gestures, and hurried mannerisms, all of which may heighten intimidations, embarrassment, fear, insecurity, and lack of trust during the examination.
- If a language interpreter is necessary, speak to the patient rather than to the interpreter; doing so enables the patient to "read" the nurse's nonverbal language.
- Avoid using metaphors and idioms unless the nurse is knowledgeable regarding language variations.

Suggested Sequence of the Physical Examination

Note

The following sequence illustrates one method to integrate all systems for a complete examination at one time. This method focuses on efficiency of time and helps protect and preserve the patient's energy. This section presents an overview of the sequence of the physical examination. Part 3 presents the details for the examination of each body system.

Examination

OVERVIEW

- Vital signs: pulse, blood pressure, respiration, temperature, and pain

- Height, weight
- Speech, cognition, mental status, interaction
- Gait, Romberg, coordination, balance

INTEGUMENT (*PATIENT SITTING*)

- Inspect and palpate all visible skin surfaces.
- Evaluate lesions (sketch them if helpful).
- Inspect hair and nails.

HEAD

- Inspect, palpate
- Cranium
- Eyes, cranial nerves (CN) II, III, IV, V, VI
- Ears, CN VIII
- Nose, CN I
- Sinuses
- Mouth, CN XII
- Throat, CN IX
- Preauricular and postauricular and occipital nodes

NECK

- Inspect, palpate, auscultate
- Carotid pulses
- Thyroid gland
- Lymph nodes
- Range of motion (ROM), CN XI
- Jugular veins

BACK

- Inspect, percuss, palpate, auscultate
- Fremitus, respiratory excursion
- Symmetry, spinal alignment
- Costovertebral angle tenderness
- Mobility

ANTERIOR TRUNK (*PATIENT SEATED AND/OR LYING*)

- Inspect the breasts.
- Auscultate breath sounds, heart sounds, carotid pulses, apical impulse (compare rate of apical impulse with radial pulse).
- Assess ROM of upper extremities.
- Palpate brachial pulses.
- Palpate the breasts, axillary, and epitrochlear lymph nodes.
- Palpate thrills, point of maximum intensity.
- With patient on left side or leaning forward, auscultate apex for murmurs.

ABDOMEN

- Inspect movement, color, contour.
- Auscultate the four quadrants.
- Auscultate for bruits over abdominal aorta, renal artery, iliac artery, and femoral artery.
- Percuss the abdomen.
- Palpate the abdomen.
- Palpate and/or percuss for bladder distention.
- Measure the size of the liver.
- Palpate the inguinal nodes, femoral pulses.
- Assess ROM of remaining joints if the patient is unable to stand.
- Palpate popliteal, dorsalis pedis, and posterior tibial pulses.

MUSCULOSKELETAL SYSTEM

- Assess weight bearing, gait, posture.
- Check extremities for edema.
- Inspect and palpate upper and lower extremities and joints for tenderness, heat, crepitus.
- Assess muscle development, symmetry, tone.
- Check ROM of lower extremities, equal length of extremities.

NEUROLOGIC SYSTEM

- Assess color, warmth, strength, ROM, gait, gross motor movement.

- Test the reflexes: Biceps, triceps, brachioradialis, patellar, achilles, plantar.
- Test balance, proprioception, fine motor movement.
- Test the cranial nerves if not previously tested.
- Test sensory perception.

GENITOURINARY SYSTEM (*PATIENT STANDING AND IN LITHOTOMY POSITION*)

- External and internal genitalia
- Pap smear
- Rectal examination
- Prostate examination

■ General Guidelines for Documentation of Findings

- Documentation of assessment is an important communication step. Without adequate recording, the assessment is limited in its use and value. Documentation helps the health-care team exchange information and prevents the patient from enduring needless repetitions. The patient's record is a confidential, consistent source of data about the patient, both baseline data and changes in condition, as well as treatments and responses.

- In addition to communication, the written medical record serves other purposes. It is a legal document, and parts of it may be admitted into evidence in court. The record can be thought of as a legal description of the patient's experience with health-care providers. A common saying in clinical settings is "if it was not charted, it was not done." Without documentation in the record, for example, the nurse may have a difficult time convincing a jury that the patient was assessed appropriately before the administration of a medication.

- The medical record also provides a source of data for audits, statistical analysis, and research. For example, a nursing quality management committee may review a series of records of discharged patients to determine the consistency of documentation of assessing venipuncture sites. Research may be conducted by evaluating the interventions recorded regarding cleansing urinary catheters of immobile patients.

Incidences of nosocomial infections can be tracked by the infection control nurse.

- Finally, patient medical records may be seen as care studies for students in the health-care field. The written chronology of a patient's experience provides students with human responses to illness. For example, the medical record may illustrate the changes in laboratory data as a patient with liver failure begins to decline.

- The system of documentation varies widely in agencies and institutions. The nurse may record data using a computer terminal at the bedside, write in a descriptive narrative in longhand, or use a series of abbreviations, symbols, and acronyms on a standardized flow sheet. Follow the appropriate form, and use only those abbreviations accepted by the agency or institution. If a narrative is required, record findings in a manner that is clear, concise, complete, accurate, and systematic.

- Examples of documentation can be found at the end of each body system section. The following guidelines may be useful in writing narratives:

  - Record all names, dates, and times completely and clearly on the correct chart.

  - Write legibly.

  - Record statements or descriptions without bias or undue interpretation. For example, if a patient accuses a nurse of following him and snooping into his affairs, the nurse should record the statements and behaviors of the patient rather than describe the patient as paranoid.

  - Avoid generalizations. Rather than "wound appears infected," make note of the color, swelling, temperature, drainage, and presence of pain.

  - Always document exceptions, abnormalities, or changes in the patient's condition. For example, any arrhythmia, bleeding, or cyanosis should be reported and documented.

  - Note normal findings in situations when abnormalities might be expected. For example, a pregnant patient with hypertension, visual disturbances, and epigastric pain could be expected to demonstrate hyperactive deep tendon reflexes. Therefore, even if the reflexes are a normal +2, this information has particular significance.

- Record changes in behavior or physical condition, especially noting full date and exact time. If the sclera are slightly jaundiced, for example, documenting and reporting this change, as well as noting its previous absence, will facilitate the medical response.
- Document as quickly as possible after the action, sign all notes, and avoid recording for others except in unusual circumstances. Keep notes until you chart them.
- In case of late additions to charting or an error, follow agency or institution policy, noting exact date and time.

Suggestions for Ease in Recording

- Record findings on the form provided by the institution (if available).
- If the institution does not have a specific form for documenting assessment data, use the nurses' notes to record the assessment, following a systematic approach (based on a specific order of systems and a specific order within each system).
- Document (record) all normal and abnormal physical findings in a clear, organized, readable, succinct, systematic manner.
- Use only abbreviations and terms accepted by the institution or agency.
- Use a capital letter at the beginning and a period at the end of each statement. Use other punctuation as needed for clarity. Complete sentences are not necessary.
- Some institutions have bedside computer terminals so that assessment data can be recorded in the patient's room as soon as possible. Written data can usually be added to the hard copy.

REMEMBER

For diagnostic, treatment, and legal reasons, it is better to record too much than too little.

PART 3

Body Organ and System Assessment

CHAPTER **5**

General Overview of Systems (with Examples)

Note and Document the Following Information about the Patient:

- *Apparent age:* Compare with stated or actual age.
- *Weight:* Note if clothing and/or shoes are included in measurements.
- *Height:* Remove the patient's shoes and use a stadiometer.
- *Arm span:* Equal to height except in older patients because of decreasing height with increasing age.
- *Vital signs:* Take blood pressure (BP) in lying, sitting, and standing positions. Repeat in other arm if elevated. Do not take BP in arm on mastectomy side or limb with dialysis access. Elevate arm to the same level as the heart.
- *Body type:* Tall, short, obese, thin, unusual body build.
- *Posture:* Straight, stooped.
- *Gait:* Fast, slow, limping, shuffling.
- *Body movements:* Mannerisms, tremors.
- *Obvious odors:* Alcohol, perfume, infection, poor hygiene.
- *Personal hygiene:* Hair, oral hygiene, nails.
- *Manner of dress:* Style, casual, hospital gown.
- *Speech:* Clear, weak, slurred, hesitant, stuttering.
- *Affect:* Flat, hostile, alert.
- *Mood and manner:* Cheerful, depressed, crying.

◤ Physical Assessment Vital Signs:

Equipment

- Thermometer, lubricant, watch with second hand, stethoscope, sphygmomanometer, gloves, disposable sheaths

Assessment of the Adult

HEALTH HISTORY

- Inquire about known temperature elevations, elevated blood pressure, pulse, and breathing problems.

TEMPERATURE

- Inquire about recent ingestion of fluids, food, or smoking within last 10 minutes.
- Secure appropriate thermometer, and shake down to 94°F (34.4°C) if mercury-in-glass type is used. Apply disposable sheath, if applicable.
- *Oral:* Place tip of thermometer near base of tongue; ask patient to close lips. Keep in place 3 minutes if using mercury-in-glass thermometer, until beeps are completed if using electronic thermometer, or until dots change color if using a disposable thermometer. Normal range is 97.5°F to 99.5°F (36°C to 38°C).
- *Rectal:* With patient in left lateral Sims' position, gently insert lubricated tip 1 to 1.5 in. Hold in place 3 minutes if using mercury-in-glass thermometer or until beeps are completed if using electronic thermometer. Normal range is 98°F to 100.5°F (37°C to 38.8°C)—usually 0.5°F to 1°F higher than oral.
- *Axillary:* With patient's arm raised, place tip of thermometer at center of axilla. Lower arm completely. Leave in place 7 to 10 minutes. Normal range is 96.5°F to 99°F (35°C to 36.8°C). Axillary: Usually 0.5°F to 1°F lower than oral.
- *Tympanic membrane:* Place clean disposable cover on the ear speculum. Gently pull pinna back. Insert speculum gently into external ear canal. Thermometer registers in seconds. Normal range is approximately the same as the oral method. 97°F to 100°F (36°C to 37.8°C).

Pulse

- *Rate:* Palpate radial pulse for 30 seconds and multiply times 2. Count for 1 full minute if irregular. Also assess for regular rhythm, strength (full, not bounding or thready), and equality (compare left and right). Normal range is 60 to 100 beats per minute.

Respiration

- *Rate:* Count breaths for 1 minute: normal range is 12 to 20 per minute. Also assess depth and rhythm and use of accessory muscles.

Blood Pressure

- Auscultate BP in sitting position over brachial artery (slightly above and inner side of antecubital space) at level of heart. Auscultate in standing and lying positions. Assess lying BP first if assessing for postural hypotension. Repeat in other arm if elevated. Do not use the arm on the side of a mastectomy or dialysis access. Based on 2 readings, 5 minutes apart, sitting in chair with feet on floor. Elevated readings confirmed in other arm. Normal systolic less than 120 mm Hg, normal diastolic less than 80 mm Hg. Prehypertension 120 to 139 mm Hg systolic, and 80 to 89 mm Hg diastolic. Hypertension 140 mm Hg or more systolic and 90 mm Hg or more diastolic.
- Blood pressure should not drop 20 mm Hg or more as the patient rises from a sitting to a standing position.

Pediatric Adaptations

Temperature

- *Rectal:* Place child prone on bed or across parent's lap. Use one arm across buttocks to restrain. Insert lubricated thermometer 0.5 to 1.0 in. Hand holding the thermometer should be braced against child's body to prevent injury.
- *Tympanic membrane:* Use ear tug to ensure accuracy. Pull pinna down and back. Explain device before approaching child, who may perceive the apparatus as a gun.

- *Ranges:*

Age	°C	°F
Children from birth to aged 1 year	99.7 to 99.4	37.7 to 37.5
Children from 1 to 3 years	99.4 to 99.0	37.5 to 37.2
Children aged 3 to 5 years	99.0 to 98.6	37.2 to 37.0
Children aged 5 to 7 years	98.6 to 98.3	37.0 to 36.8
Children aged 7 to 9 years	98.3 to 98.1	36.8 to 36.7
Children aged 10 years and older	97.8	36.6

PULSE

- Use apical rate, not radial.
- *Ranges of heart rates:*

	Beats Per Minute (BPM)
Children at birth	80 to 160
Children from birth to aged 3 months	80 to 180
Children aged 3 months to Children aged 2 years	80 to 150
Children aged 2 to 10 years	70 to 110
Children aged 10 years and older	55 to 90

RESPIRATION

- Most accurate rate is counted when child is sleeping. Watch movement of the abdomen of infant.
- *Ranges of respiratory rates:*

	Breaths Per Minute
Children at birth	30 to 40
Children aged 1 year	20 to 40
Children aged 2 years	20 to 30
Children aged 5 years	20 to 25
Children aged 10 years	17 to 22
Children aged 15 years	15 to 20

BLOOD PRESSURE

- *Ranges:*

Age	Systolic/Diastolic (mm Hg)
Children aged 1 month	86/54
Children aged 1 year	96/65
Children aged 4 years	99/65
Children aged 6 years	100/60
Children aged 8 years	105/60
Children aged 10 years	110/60
Children aged 12 years	115/60
Children aged 14 years	118/60
Children aged 16 years	120/65

Geriatric Adaptations

TEMPERATURE

- Tympanic membrane thermometer is ideal because it is quick and safe.
- Oral method may not be accurate if the person cannot keep the mouth closed for the required length of time.
- Rectal or axillary method should not be used unless absolutely necessary.
- Note that older adults may remain afebrile during an infection because of a lower baseline temperature, a decreased metabolic rate, and a decreased immune response.

PULSE RATE

- No major changes in old age but may decrease in persons aged 85 and older.

RESPIRATION

- Depth may decrease and rate may increase.
- If you experience difficulty counting, observe and count the rise and fall of the abdomen.

BLOOD PRESSURE

- Normal systolic and diastolic BP are the same as in other adults. Pulse pressure (systolic-diastolic) may increase.
  See Table 5–1 for variations in normal vital signs for the adult.

Table 5-1

Variations in Normal Vital Signs for the Adult

	Oral Temperature in (Fahrenheit)	Pulse (BPM)	Respiration (Breath Perminute)	Blood Pressure (mmHg)
Adult	98.6°	80	16	<120/80
Older adult	96.8°	70	16	<120/80

Individuals older than 55 have a 90% lifetime risk for developing hypertension. A systolic BP of 120 mm Hg or a diastolic BP of 80 to 89 mm Hg should be considered prehypertensive and require health promoting lifestyle modifications.

Data for this table were compiled from the following sources:
Kozier, B, Erb, G, Berman, A, Snyder, SJ (eds.): Fundamentals of Nursing, ed. 7.
Pearson Prentice Hall, Upper Saddle River, NJ, 2004, p. 485.
Potter, PA, and Perry, AG: Fundamentals of Nursing, ed. 5. Mosby, St Louis, MO, 2001, pp. 730–731.
Department of Health and Human Services, National Heart, Lung, and Blood Institute: Seventh Report of the Joint National Committee on the Prevention, Detection, Evaluation, and Treatment of High Blood Pressure, NIH Pub No. 03–5233 (electronic version). National Heart, Lung, Blood Institute Information Center, Bethesda, Md, May 2003 retrieved March 17, 2004 from http://www.nhlbi.nih.gov/guidelines/hypertension/express.pdf

Physical Assessment: Pain

Pain perception and expression is based on many factors such as age, ethnicity, gender, culture, and experience with previous pain. Eleven characteristics to assess are location, quality, quantity, radiation, associated manifestations, timing, alienating factors, setting, aggravating factors, meaning, and impact.

Rating scales have been developed for assessing pain for adults and children.

Pediatric Scale Used for Those Persons Aged 3 Years and Older.

Brief word instructions: Point to each face using the words to describe the pain intensity. Ask the child to choose the face that best describes his or her own pain; record the appropriate number.

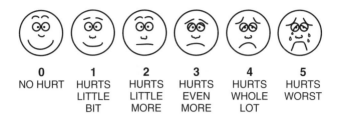

Figure 5-1 Wong-Baker FACES Pain Rating Scale. (From Wong D L, Hockenberry-Eaton, M, Wilson D., Winkelstein M.L., Schwartz P: *Wong's Essentials of Pediatric Nursing*, ed.6, St. Louis, mo., 2001, p. 1301. Copyrighted by Mosby, Inc. Reprinted by permission.)

Adult and Geriatric

A common, easy-to-use pain scale for adults and older adults is simply to ask them to verbally rate their pain from 0 as no pain to 10 as the worst possible pain. A vertical scale works better than a horizontal scale because 0 is the lowest number and 10 is the highest number. See Figure 5–2 Pain Rating Scale for Older Adults.

◼ Physical Assessment—Body Weight

Introduction

- A healthy weight is a range of body weight based on age, height, and gender that is statistically related to good health. Being above or below that range increases the risk of health problems, or decreases the likelihood of good health. Both underweight and overweight ranges may reflect energy imbalance in a patient, with total caloric expenditure unequal to total energy intake.

- Underweight is generally accepted as being below 10 percent of ideal body weight (IBW) and is indicative of malnutrition or inadequate energy intake.

- Overweight is defined as 10 to 20 percent above IBW and is usually the result of increased energy intake coupled with decreased energy expenditure.

Table 5-2

FLACC NONVERBAL PAIN SCALE

Categories	Scoring		
	0	1	2
Face (F)	No particular expression or smile, eye contact, and interest in surroundings	Occasional grimace or frown, withdrawn, disinterested, worried look to face, eyebrows lowered, eyes partially closed, cheeks raised, mouth pursed	Frequent to constant frown, clenched jaw, quivering chin, deep furrows on forehead, eyes closed, mouth opened, deep lines around nose/lips
Legs (L)	Normal position or relaxed	Uneasy, restless, tense, increased tone, rigidity, intermittent flexion/extension of limbs	Kicking or legs drawn up, hypertonicity, exaggerated flexion/extension of limbs, tremors
Activity (A)	Lying quietly, normal position, moves easily and freely	Squirming, shifting back and forth, tense, hesitant to move, guarding, pressure on body part	Arched, rigid, or jerking, fixed position, rocking, side-to-side head movement, rubbing of body part
Cry (C)	No cry/moan (awake or asleep)	Moans or whimpers, occasional cries, sighs, occasional complaint	Crying steadily, screams, sobs, moans, grunts, frequent complaints
Consolability (C)	Calm, content, relaxed, does not require consoling	Reassured by occasional touching, hugging, or 'talking to'; distractible	Difficult to console or comfort

Each of the five categories (F) Face, (L) Legs, (A) Activity, (C) Cry, (C) Consolability is scored from 0–2, which results in a total score between zero and 10. The FLACC Pain Scale can be used with infant and pediatric patients from birth to three years, cognitively impaired patients, and those patients unable to use other scales. The previous words that are bolded apply to all patients EXCEPT infant and pediatric patients.

FLACC—Assess the patient in each area—total the score—evaluate the total using the 0 to 10 pain scale parameters.

Merkel S, Voepel-Lewis T & Malviya S. Pain control, pain assessment in infants and young children: the FLACC Scale: A behavioral tool to measure pain in young children. American Journal of Nursing 102(10):55–6, 58, 2002.

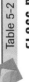

10	Worst possible pain
9	
8	
7	
6	
5	Moderate pain
4	
3	
2	
1	Least pain
0	No pain

Figure 5-2 Pain rating scale for older adults

Assessment of Healthy Weight

- The following assessment methods and body weight criteria categorize healthy weight, underweight, and overweight (obesity in adults, pediatrics, and geriatric patients).

  ADULT AND GERIATRIC ADAPTATIONS DETERMINING A HEALTHY OR IDEAL BODY WEIGHT (IBW)

- Hamwi Method — Calculations available.

  Source: Nutrition and Your Health: Dietary Guidelines for Americans. ed. 3. Washington, DC: U.S. Depts of Agriculture and Health and Human Services: 1990 Home and Garden Bulletin No. 232.

  Reference: Hamwi GJ: Changing dietary concepts. In Danowski, TS (ed): Diabetes Mellitus: Diagnosis and Treatment, Vol. 1. American Diabetes Association, Inc; New York; 1964; p. 73–78.

- Healthy Weight Chart (see Appendix O) Source: Report of the Dietary Guidelines Advisory Committee on the Dietary Guidelines for Americans, 2000, p. 3. Contact: *http://www.usda.gov/cnpp/Pubs/DG2000/*

- Body Mass Index (BMI) (see Appendix O) is a weight to height ratio (kg/m^2) that is used as an indicator for classifications of underweight (18.5 or less), ideal or healthy weight (18.5 to 24.9), overweight (25 to 29.9), and obesity (30 or more) (see Appendix O) Source: Report of the Dietary Guidelines Advisory Committee on the Dietary Guidelines for Americans, 2000, p. 3. Contact:*http://www.usda.gov/cnpp/Pubs/DG2000/*

PEDIATRIC ADAPTATIONS (SEE APPENDIX O)

- Length-for-age and Weight-for-age percentiles and/or Head circumference-for-age and Weight-for-length percentiles are gender and age specific for persons from birth to 36 months, which assess rate of growth and development. Source: Developed by the National Center for Health Statistics in collaboration with the National Center for Chronic Disease Prevention and Health Promotion, 2000. Contact: *http://www.cdc.gov/growthcharts*

- BMI-for-Age percentiles are gender and age specific for children and adolescents and is used primarily to assess rate of growth and development. BMI criteria for persons aged 2 to 20 years denote underweight, at risk for overweight, and overweight. Source: Developed by the National Center for Health Statistics in collaboration with the National Center for Chronic Disease Prevention and Health Promotion, 2000. Contact:*http://www.cdc.gov/growthcharts*

GERIATRIC ADAPTATIONS

- BMI (see Appendix O) Contact:*http://www.nhlbi.nih.gov/guidelines/obesity/bmi_tbl.pdf* Source: Adapted from Clinical Guidelines on the Identification, Evaluation, and Treatment of Overweight and Obesity in Adults: The Evidence Report. National Heart, Lung, and Blood Institute, in cooperation with the National Institute of Diabetes and Digestive and Kidney Diseases Contact: *http://www. nhlbi.nih.gov/guidelines/obesity/ob_home.htm*

- Average Height and Weight for Persons Aged 65 Years and Older Source: Adapted from the Average Height and Weight for Persons Aged 65 Years and Older; Morrison's Manual of Clinical Nutrition Management, 2003: JAMA 172:658, 1960.

Overweight and Obesity

Introduction—Overweight and Obesity in Adults

- Obesity is the most common chronic disease of the industrialized world, and is becoming increasingly problematic in developing countries as well. An estimated 97 million adults in the U.S. are overweight or obese, a condition that substantially raises the risk of morbidity from coronary heart disease, type 2 diabetes, hypertension, stroke, gallbladder disease, osteoarthritis, and certain cancers. Higher body weights are also associated with increases in all-cause mortality. Overweight and obesity are the second leading causes of preventable deaths in the U.S. today and pose a major public health challenge.

- Obesity is a multifaceted problem involving physiologic, psychologic, and cultural factors—all of which are resistant to current therapeutic efforts. Metabolic and glandular disorders, heredity, basal metabolic rate, and body type all influence the development of obesity. Although the exact mechanism that causes obesity is not known, the main factor appears to be an energy imbalance attributable to overeating combined with inadequate levels of physical activity.

Assessment

- Overweight in adults is defined as a BMI of 25 to 29.9 kg/m^2 and obesity in adults as a BMI of 30 or more kg/m^2 (see Appendix O). Source: Adapted from the Practical Guide: Identification, Evaluation, and Treatment of Overweight and Obesity in Adults; developed by the North American Association for the Study of Obesity (NAASO) and the National Heart, Lung, and Blood Institute (NHLBI), 2000. Contact:*http://www/nhlbi.nih.gov/guidelines/obesity/practgde. htm.*

- When assessing a patient's weight status and associated disease risk, both BMI and waist circumference are determined. BMI and waist circumference are interrelated. Waist circumference is the most practical tool to evaluate a patient's abdominal fat before and during weight loss treatment. Fat located in the abdominal region is associated with a greater health risk than peripheral fat.

- Gender-specific cut points can be used to identify increased risk for the development of obesity-associated disease in most adults, with a BMI of 25 to 34.9 kg/m². These categories denote relative risk, not absolute risk—that is, relative to risk at normal weight.

- For people who are considered obese or those who are overweight, the guidelines recommend weight loss. Even a small weight loss (10 percent of current weight) will help to lower risk of developing diseases associated with obesity.

Pediatric Adaptations

- The occurrence of overweight and obesity in children has tripled in the past 30 years, and is now estimated that one in five children in the U.S. is overweight. Obesity rates in children have risen as well. Based on current statistics from the Centers for Disease Control (CDC) and Prevention, approximately 13 percent of children aged 6 to 11 and 14 percent of adolescents aged 12 to 19 are considered overweight. Increases in the prevalence of overweight are also being seen in younger children, including preschoolers.

- Both short-term and long-term effects of overweight on health are concerns because of the negative psychologic and health consequences in childhood. Compared with normal-weight peers, overweight children are more likely to become obese adults, with an increased risk for a number of chronic diseases associated with obesity. Research shows that 60 percent of overweight children aged 5 to 10 years have at least one heart disease risk factor. Obese children are about 50 percent more likely to develop insulin resistance, and often preceded adult-onset type 2 diabetes.

- Contributors to childhood overweight and obesity include:
  - Food choices—diets higher in calories and lower in fruits and vegetables
  - Physical activity vs. sedentary activity—less physical activity and more time spent participating in activities such as watching TV results in less energy expenditure

- Parental eating and physical activity habits—parents with poor nutritional habits and who lead sedentary lifestyles role model these behaviors for their children
- Parental obesity and genetics—children of obese parents are more likely to be overweight
- Eating patterns—skipping meals or failure to maintain a regular eating schedule can result in increased food intake.

ASSESSMENT

- Childhood overweight and obesity are determined by calculating BMI that is plotted on the CDC's BMI-for-Age growth charts for children of the same age and sex. Children with a BMI between the 85th to 95th percentile for age and sex are classified as risks for overweight, and children who have a BMI at or above the 95th percentile are considered overweight. Parents whose children fall in the overweight category should make an appointment with their pediatrician or family physician to discuss whether treatment is warranted.
- CDC's BMI-for-Age growth charts (see Appendix O) Source: Developed by the National Center for Health Statistics in collaboration with the National Center for Chronic Disease Prevention and Health Promotion, 2000 Contact.*http:// www.cdc.gov/growthcharts.*

Weight Management Goals

- Overall goals of weight loss and management include (1) preventing further weight gain, (2) reducing body weight, and (3) maintaining a lower body weight over the long term.
- Recommendations for reaching and maintaining a healthy weight include following a sensible eating plan and engaging in regular physical activity. Safe and effective weight-loss programs should include the following goals:
  - Healthy eating plans that reduce calories but do not rule out specific foods or food groups
  - Regular physical activity and/or exercise regimen
  - Tips on healthy behavior changes that also consider cultural needs

- Progressive and steady weight loss of approximately three-fourths to 2 lbs/week, and not more than 3 lbs/week
- Medical care if patient is planning to lose weight by following a special diet such as a very-low-calorie diet (LCD)
- Plan of long-term weight management program to keep the weight off

Tips for Weight Loss and Weight Management

- **Dietary therapy** with a deficit of 500 to 1,000 kcal/day should be an integral part of a weight loss program. Depending on the patient's risk status and physician's advice, the LCD may be recommended for weight loss in overweight and obese individuals.

  - **Initial goal of weight loss therapy** is to reduce body weight by approximately 10 percent from baseline. A reasonable timeline for a 10 percent reduction in body weight is 6 months of therapy.

    - Overweight patients with BMIs of 27 to 35 kg/m^2: a decrease of 300 to 500 kcal/day will result in weight losses of approximately one-half to 1 lb/week and a 10 percent loss in 6 months.

    - Obese patients with BMIs over 35 kg/m^2: a decrease of 500 to 1,000 kcal/day will lead to weight losses of approximately 1 to 2 lb/week and a 10 percent weight loss in 6 months.

  - **If more weight loss is needed after 6 months,** further adjustment of decreased caloric intake and physical activity regimens can be outlined.

- **Physical activity** is recommended as part of a comprehensive weight loss therapy and weight control program because it (1) contributes to greater energy expenditure and weight loss, (2) may decrease abdominal fat, (3) increases cardiorespiratory fitness, and (4) helps to maintain long-term weight. Recommendations to patients should include:

  - For most individuals, exercise should be initiated slowly, and the intensity should be increased gradually.

- Exercise can be done all at one time or intermittently over the day.
- Choose physical activities that fit in with daily routines, recreational or structured exercise programs, or both.
- Initially, moderate levels of physical activity for 30 to 45 minutes—3 to 5 days/week—should be encouraged.
- All adults should set a long-term goal to accumulate at least 30 minutes or more of moderate-intensity physical activity on all days of the week.
- Children and teens need at least 60 minutes of physical activity daily.
- Older persons also need to be physically active and should engage in moderate physical activity for at least 30 minutes most days of the week, preferably daily. Adding activities to strengthen muscles will improve flexibility.
- Patients should consult with a health-care provider before starting a new vigorous physical activity plan if they have a chronic health problem, or if they are over 40 (men) or 50 (women) years of age.

- **Weight maintenance**—after successful weight loss, the likelihood of weight loss maintenance is enhanced by the combined intervention of diet therapy, physical activity, and behavior modification, and can be continued indefinitely.

CHAPTER **6**

Integument

History

Note

A brief review of the essential components of the history is included at the beginning of each system. In many clinical situations, the nurse will be concentrating primarily on one or more systems, rather than a total, integrated health assessment.

Adult

- Previous skin diseases
- Years of exposure to sun, use of tanning beds, and other environmental factors
- Recent change in a wart or mole
- Any sore that has not healed
- Rashes, lesions, abrasions, bruises
- Tick bites
- Adverse effects of medications
- Allergies, seasonal or climatic effects
- Recent changes in hair growth, distribution
- Recent changes in nails (e.g., ridges, thickening, color bands)
- Recent changes in sensation of pain, heat, cold
- Thyroid, endocrine, and circulatory disorders

Pediatric

Infants
- Type of diaper and diaper cream used
- Method and products used for bath
- Rashes, lesions, bruises
- Injuries

(Continued on following page)

Children
- Injury history related to play (e.g., abrasions, cuts)
- Signs of abuse:
  - Injury is not congruent with adult's description of incident or developmental level of child
  - History of injury is not consistent with assessment
  - Delay in seeking care for a significant injury
  - Bruises or welts on areas of the body not injured during normal play, such as the face, lips, mouth, and lower back
  - Injuries with an identifiable shape such as a shoe, belt buckle, or circumferential; or with a sharp boundary and no splatter marks
  - Burns on the palms or soles
- Allergies
- Acne, eczema; include onset, treatment
- Recent exposure to a communicable disease

- History of skin cancers or other chronic skin conditions
- Excessive dryness, itching
- Increased bruising tendency
- Assess for signs of abuse, such as bruises about the face or ears, scars, lesions, or any kind of trauma
- Increased healing time
- Chronic, long-term sun exposure
- Marks (excoriation, redness, trauma)
- Temperature changes in skin
- Nail texture changes
- Frequency of bathing and products used for bathing

(Continued on following page)

General Considerations

- Use of home remedies or local applications of any kind on skin
- Occupational hazards (e.g., skin contact materials, radiation, abnormal lighting)
- Care of papules or minor lesions (squeezing or picking)
- Care of excess hair (shaving, plucking)
- Excessive dryness, itching
- Use of lotions, creams, oils, and other skin lubricants
- Use of special hair products
- Use of bleaching creams and other skin-lightening or tanning agents
- Increased bruising tendency
- Increased healing time

Equipment

- 6-in transparent ruler measured in centimeters as well as inches
- Penlight or flashlight
- Gloves

Patient Preparation

- Have patient sit and stand for total exposure of skin.
- Keep patient warm.
- Maintain complete privacy.

Physical Assessment: Skin

Adult

Steps	Normal and/or Common Findings	Significant Deviations
Inspection		
• *Color:* Note symmetry, shade	Pink, light brown, dark brown, ruddy, coffee, chloasma, vitiligo	Pale, cyanotic, jaundiced, sallow
• *Lesions:* Note size, location, shape, color	Nevi, scars, keloids, especially in dark pigmented skin (Fig. 6-1), striae	Tracks, varicosities, tick bites (whitened center with red circle around it)
• *Erythema:* Note location, size, blanching	None	
• *Lesions:* Note type, morphology, location, size, shape, grouping or arrangement, exudate	Macules	Papule, nodule, tumor, wheal, vesicle, bulla, pustule, erosion, excoriation, fissure, ulcer, scale, petechia, purpura, ecchymosis (Table 6–1)
Smell		
• Odors	Cigarette smoke, perspiration	Alcohol, acetone, foul odors
Palpation		
• Temperature	Warm, cool	Hot, cold
• Turgor for degree (Figs. 6-2 and 6-3)	Rebounds instantly	Tented for greater than 5 seconds
• Degree of moisture	Dry	Damp, clammy
• Texture	Smooth, even	Rough
• Lesions or lumps for pain, depth, size if not visible	None	Pain

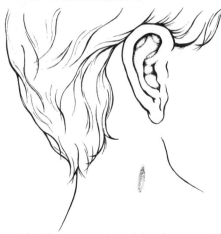

Figure 6-1 Keloid lesion on neck: nodular, firm area of hyperplastic scar tissue from previous surgery and/or trauma.

Table 6-1

Types of Skin Lesions

Lesion	Size (cm)	Description
Primary Lesions		
Macule	<1	Flat, circumscribed, varied in color
Papule	<1	Elevated, firm, solid
Nodule	1<2	Elevated, firm, solid
Tumor	>2	Elevated, firm, solid
Wheal	Varied	Transient, irregular, edematous
Vesicle	<1	Elevated, serous fluid filled
Bulla	>1	Elevated, serous fluid filled
Pustule	Varied	Elevated, purulent fluid filled
Secondary Lesions		
Erosion	Varied	Moist epidermal depression; follows rupture of vesicle, bulla
Excoriation	Varied	Crusted epidermal abrasion
Fissure	Varied	Red, linear dermal break
Ulcer	Varied	Red dermal depression; exudate
Scale	Varied	Flaky, irregular, white to silver
Petechia	<0.5	Flat, red to purple
Purpura	>0.5	Flat, red to purple
Ecchymosis	Varied	Dark red to dark blue, painful

🔲 Physical Assessment: Hair

Adult

Steps	Normal and/or Common Findings	Significant Deviations
Inspection		
• Color	Black, brown, blond, red, gray, white	
• Quantity	Thick, thin, sparse	Patchy, none
• Distribution for presence, symmetry of body hair	Varies	Alopecia, marginal alopecia, hirsutism, absence on lower limbs
• General condition	Combed, clean	Dirty, uncombed, matted
Palpation		
• Texture	Coarse, fine, curly, oily, dry	Brittle

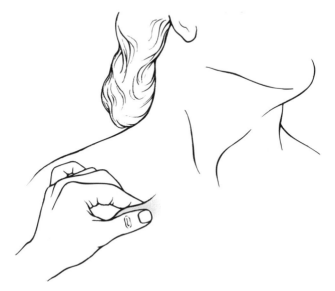

Figure 6-2 Testing skin turgor: adult.

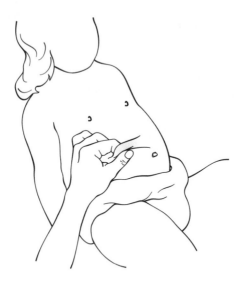

Figure 6-3 Testing skin turgor: child.

Physical Assessment: Nails

Adult

Steps	Normal and/or Common Findings	Significant Deviations
Inspection		
• Plate for color	Pink, light brown	Blue, black
• Cuticle	Smooth	Edema, erythema, exudate
• Shape	Curved	Clubbed, flattened (see also Fig. 13-1)
• Configuration (Fig. 6-4)	Longitudinal ridges	Transverse depressions or ridges, pits
• General condition	Clean, neat	Unkempt, dirty
Palpation		
• Consistency	Firm	Boggy, brittle

SPOON NAIL (KOILONYCHIA)

SPLINTER HEMORRHAGES

ONYCHOLYSIS

PARONYCHIA

TRANSVERSE GROOVING
(BEAU'S LINES)

Figure 6-4 Abnormal nail conditions.

■ Physical Assessment: Skin

Pediatric Adaptations

INFANT

Steps	Normal and/or Common Findings	Significant Deviations
Inspection • Color	Usually reflects a lighter shade of parents' skin color at birth; reddened to pink, acrocyanosis,* mongolian spots, harlequin sign, stork bite, mottling*	Pallor, physiologic jaundice, nevus flammeus, cyanosis, purpura, multiple bruises, lesions that may be inconsistent with history

(Continued on following page)

(Continued)

Steps	Normal and/or Common Findings	Significant Deviations
Inspection (Continued)		
• Texture	Smooth, soft; vernix in creases if term*	Peeling
• Lesions	Milia; forceps marks on head*	Capillary hemangioma, erythema toxicum, blisters
• Integrity	Intact	Openings, clefts especially on spine, head
• Palmar, sole creases for number, pattern	Multiple creases at term	Few to absent creases; simian line
Palpation		
• Turgor on abdomen	Instant recoil	Tenting
		Cafe au lait spots greater than 5 mm
• Lesions for size, shape, consistency		Pitting edema or periorbital edema
* Newborn only		

Physical Assessment: Hair

Pediatric Adaptations

INFANT

Steps	Normal and/or Common Findings	Significant Deviations
Inspection		
• General condition	Clean; cradle cap, lanugo*	Bald spot on back of head
		Hair tuft on spine
* Newborn only		

🔲 Physical Assessment: Nails

Pediatric Adaptations

INFANT

Steps	Normal and/or Common Findings	Significant Deviations
Inspection • Size • Shape • Color	Thin; may be long; easily cyanotic to pink	Clubbing

🔲 Physical Assessment: Skin

Pediatric Adaptations

CHILD

Steps	Normal and/or Common Findings	Significant Deviations
Inspection • Color • Common diseases	Yellowish cast from eating yellow vegetables Ringworm, impetigo, scabies	Multiple bruises, burns; ashen gray in dark-skinned persons Varicella, candidiasis

🔲 Physical Assessment: Hair

Pediatric Adaptations

CHILD

Steps	Normal and/or Common Findings	Significant Deviations
Inspection • Foreign bodies	Color may darken and thicken	Head lice, nits, ticks, alopecia, pubic hair on child less than age 9

📥 Physical Assessment: Skin

Pediatric Adaptations

ADOLESCENT

Steps	Normal and/or Common Findings	Significant Deviations
Inspection • Sebaceous glands	Oily, acne, comedones	Pitting, scarring

📥 Physical Assessment: Hair

Pediatric Adaptations

ADOLESCENT

Steps	Normal and/or Common Findings	Significant Deviations
• *Body hair:* Note amount, pattern, texture	Increases in amount; coarseness; progresses toward adult fullness and texture	Sparse, scanty, fine, patchy

📥 Physical Assessment: Skin

Geriatric Adaptations

Steps	Normal and/or Common Findings	Significant Deviations
Inspection • Color	*Lentigo:* Back of hands, arms, face	Erythema; bruises (head and trunk more significant than arms or legs as possible signs of abuse)

(Continued on following page)

Steps	Normal and/or Common Findings	Significant Deviations
• Temperature	Cool	Uneven, asymmetrical, very cold
• Moisture	Dry, scaling, decreased perspiration	Cracked, fissured, marked flaking
• Texture	Thinning, transparent	
• *Turgor:* Check on forehead, chest or abdomen (see Fig. 6-2)	Wrinkling, decreased subcutaneous fat, sagging	Extended tenting, excessive sagging (weight loss)
• Lesions (Fig. 6-5)	Cherry angiomas, seborrheic keratosis, acrochordons, purpura	Actinic keratosis, basal cell carcinoma, squamous cell carcinoma, herpes zoster, pressure ulcers (Fig. 6-6 and Table 6-2)

■ Physical Assessment: Hair

Geriatric Adaptations

Steps	Normal and/or Common Findings	Significant Deviations
Inspection		
• Color	Loss of pigment greater than age 50	
• Quantity	Decreased body hair, hirsutism, decreased hair on lower extremities, thinning of hair on head	Unusual alopecia, asymmetrical

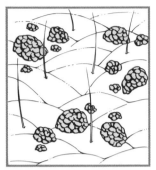

A. CHERRY ANGIOMA.   **B.** ACTINIC KERATOSIS.

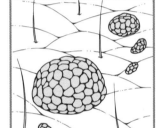

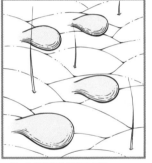

C. SEBORRHEIC KERATOSIS.   **D.** ACROCHORDON.

Figure 6-5 Common skin changes in older adults. (*A*) Cherry angioma. (*B*) Actinic keratosis. (*C*) Seborrheic keratosis. (*D*) Acrochordon.

◼ Physical Assessment: Nails

Geriatric Adaptations

Steps	Normal and/or Common Findings	Significant Deviations
Inspection • Texture	Ridges, longitudinal splitting, thickening, decreased growth	

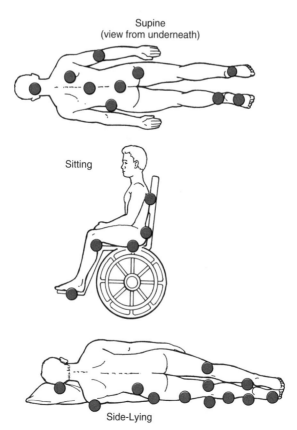

Supine
(view from underneath)

Sitting

Side-Lying

Figure 6-6 Body prominences prone to pressure ulcers.

Table 6-2

Stages of Pressure Ulcers

The National Pressure Ulcer Advisory Panel has classified pressure
   ulcers into four stages:

Stage I   Nonblanchable erythema of intact skin.
Stage II   Partial-thickness skin loss involving the epidermis or
                dermis.

(Continued on following page)

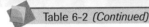
Table 6-2 (Continued)

Stages of Pressure Ulcers

Stage III   Full-thickness skin loss involving subcutaneous tissue that may extend to, but not through, the underlying fascia.

Stage IV   Deeper, full-thickness lesions extending into muscle or bone.

Eschar   Ulcers covered by eschar (hard necrotic tissue) are unstageable and usually represent ulcers of at least a stage III.

(Source: Clinical Practice Guideline: Treatment of Pressure Ulcers. U.S. Department of Health and Human Services, Public Health Service, Agency for Health Care Policy and Research, Rockville, Md. December 1994, vol. 15.)

▧ Physical Assessment: Skin

Cultural Adaptations

Steps	Normal and/or Common Findings	Significant Deviations
Inspection		
• *Color:* Changes best observed in sclera, conjunctivae, oral mucosa, tongue, lips, nail beds, palms, soles (Table 6–3)	Ranges from deep black to light brown to olive and yellow overtones	Edema causes dark skin to appear lighter
	Wrinkled skin areas appear darker (knees, elbows)	*Pallor:* Brown skin becomes yellow; black skin becomes ashen gray
	Calloused areas appear yellow (palms, soles)	Cyanosis noted in nail beds, conjunctivae, palms, soles
	Dark-skinned clients may have lips with blue hue	Petechiae noted in conjunctivae and oral mucosa
	Oral mucosa darker pigmentation in gums, cheeks, borders of tongue	Signs of sickle cell disease: Jaundice, pallor, chronic leg ulcers
	Keloid scar formation after surgery, tattoos, and cosmetic piercing	
Palpation	Smooth	Rashes may not be detected by inspection
	Cool	Erythema not easily detected by inspection

Table 6-3

Assessment of Skin Color

Characteristic	White or Light-Skinned Person	Dark-Skinned Person
Pallor		
Vasoconstriction present	Skin takes on white hue, which is color of collagen fibers in subcutaneous connective tissue	Skin loses underlying red tones; brown-skinned person appears yellow-brown; black-skinned person appears ashen gray
		Mucous membranes, lips, nailbeds pale or gray; skin appears yellow-brown or ashen gray
Erythema, Inflammation		
Cutaneous vasodilation	Skin is red	Palpate for increased warmth of skin, edema, tightness, or induration of skin; streaking and redness difficult to assess
Cyanosis		
Hypoxia of tissues	Bluish tinges of skin, especially in earlobes, as well as in lips, oral mucosa, and nail beds	Lips, tongue, conjunctivae, palms, soles of feet are pale or ashen gray
		Apply light pressure to create pallor; in cyanosis tissue color returns slowly by spreading from periphery to the center

(Continued on following page)

Table 6-3 *(Continued)*

Assessment of Skin Color

Characteristic	White or Light-Skinned Person	Dark-Skinned Person
Ecchymosis		
Deoxygenated blood seeps from broken blood vessel into subcutaneous tissue	Skin changes color from purple-blue to yellow-green to yellow	Oral mucous membrane or conjunctivae will show color changes from purple-blue to yellow-green to yellow Obtain history of trauma and discomfort Note swelling and induration
Petechiae		
Intradermal or submucosal bleeding	Round, pinpoint purplish-red spots are present on skin	Oral mucosa or conjunctivae show purplish-red spots if person has black skin
Jaundice		
Accumulated bilirubin in tissues	Yellow color in skin, mucous membranes, and sclera of eyes Light-colored stools and dark urine often occur	Sclera of eyes, oral mucous membranes, palms of hand, and soles of feet have yellow discoloration

*(**Source:** Adapted from Murray, RB, and Zentner, JP: Nursing Assessment and Health Promotion Strategies through the Life Span, ed 7. Prentice Hall, Upper Saddle River, NJ, 2001, 51, with permission.)*

📖 Physical Assessment: Hair

Cultural Adaptations

Steps	Normal and/or Common Findings	Significant Deviations
Inspection		
• Color	Wide variation from light brown to deep black	
• Quantity	Thick, thin, sparse	Thinning
• Distribution	Present on scalp, lower face, nares, ears, axillae, anterior chest around nipples, arms, legs, back of hands and feet, back, buttocks	Alopecia
• Texture	*Scalp:* Fine or coarse *Body:* Fine *Pubic* and *axillary:* Coarse	Brittle
• Lesions	Small, inflamed pustules near hair follicles	Scars or burns from heat or chemicals

📖 Physical Assessment: Nails

Cultural Adaptations

Steps	Normal and/or Common Findings	Significant Deviations
Inspection		
• Color	Pigment deposits in nail beds in dark-skinned clients	

📖 Diagnostic Tests
• Refer to physician for biopsy of suspicious lesions

📖 Possible Nursing Diagnoses
• Infection, risk for
• Injury, risk for

- Tissue integrity, impaired
- Trauma, risk for
- Skin integrity, impaired
- Skin integrity, risk for impaired
- Self-care deficit, feeding, bathing/hygiene, dressing/grooming, toileting
- Body image disturbance
- Self-esteem disturbance
- Unilateral neglect

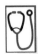

Clinical Alert

- Report all suspicious lesions.
- Report suspicious bruising, especially around the mouth, eyes, or ears or on the chest (could be signs of abuse).
- Note problems with cleanliness, grooming.

■ Sample Documentation

Skin bilaterally pale pink and elastic, with no varicosities, ecchymoses, edema, or erythema. Multiple striae present along lower abdomen and medial aspects of breasts. Abundant maculae scattered across nose, cheeks, and backs of ears. Raised white scar, 2 cm in diameter, on upper outer aspect of left arm. Skin on extremities symmetrical, cool, and dry. No noticeable odors. Hair thick, fine, light brown, and distributed normally on head. No hirsutism or hair loss noted. Nails slightly curved, firm, with no ridges or pits. Nail beds pink. No clubbing.

■ Patient and Family Education and Home Health Notes

General Considerations

- Tanned skin is damaged skin.
- Avoid exposure to sun as much as possible especially between 10:00 a.m. and 4:00 p.m. daylight savings time (9:00 a.m. to 3:00 p.m., standard time). Centers for

(Continued on following page)

Disease Control and Prevention http://www.cdc.gov/ Choose YourCover/qanda.htm#when

- When outdoors:
  - Seek shade.
  - Wear a wide-brimmed hat, long-sleeved shirt, and long pants.
  - Wear wraparound sunglasses that provide 100% ultraviolet (UV) protection.
  - Use a broad spectrum (UVA and UVB) sunscreen and lip balm with a sun protection factor (SPF) of at least 15. Check the expiration date on the sunscreen. Sunscreens without expiration dates have a maximum shelf life of 3 years.
  - Apply sunscreen according to the manufacturer's directions and reapply frequently.
- Use sun protection whether in shade or the day is cloudy.
- Use artificial tanning products cautiously.
- Do not use tanning beds.
- Avoid direct exposure to the sun, especially if using skin lightening creams.

Adult

- Prevent clothing from irritating moles, warts, and other lesions.
- Do total self-assessment of skin monthly.
- Do not push cuticle back from nail surface.

Pediatric

Infant

- Teach parents to avoid sun exposure for infants younger than 6 months of age; after 6 months of age, follow general considerations.
- Teach parents that preventing sunburn during childhood reduces the lifetime risk of developing melanoma.

(Continued on following page)

- Teach parents about general and individual variations from normal.
- Lower water heater thermometer temperature to 110° F (43.33°C).
- Test bathwater temperature before placing baby in bath.
- Instruct parents in cleansing of and caring for skin; use mild soap, rinse well, use oil only if very dry, and do not use powders. Wash scalp and fontanels.
- Clip nails when infant is asleep or quiet.
- Change diapers frequently.
- When changing diapers, cleanse from pubis to anus.

Adolescent

- Wash face with nondeodorant soap and water 2 to 3 times daily if skin is oily.
- Do not pick acne pustules.
- Continue to stress use of sunscreens.

Geriatric

- Use soap sparingly and rinse well.
- Avoid using harsh deodorant or perfumed soaps.
- Bathe 5 to 7 times a week using tepid water rather than hot water.
- Do not use alcohol or powder on skin.
- Apply a lanolin-containing emollient after bathing (while skin is still moist) to help retain moisture absorbed while bathing.
- Avoid bath oils because they can increase the risk of falls in the tub.
- Use room humidifiers or place pitcher of water over heaters to increase moisture in the air.
- Avoid wearing rough fabrics next to the skin. Wear cotton underpants.
- Keep feet and areas between toes clean and dry.
- Use manicure stick rather than metal file to clean nails.

(Continued on following page)

- Diabetics must be very meticulous with foot care (inspecting feet daily, performing foot care carefully, and having toenails cut and/or cleaned by a health-care professional).
- Patients restricted to bed must be repositioned frequently (at least every 2 hours). Position changes need not be drastic; a slight change is often adequate. Bony prominences must be well padded.
- Patients restricted to wheelchair must shift their position every 15 to 30 minutes.
- Incontinent patients must practice meticulous skin care, changing absorbent product as soon as soiled, cleansing skin well after each incontinent episode, making use of moisture barrier creams, using only absorbent pads at night to allow air to reach skin, and using external collection devices.
- Refer patient to podiatrist if unable to safely trim and clean toenails.
- Prevent prolonged pressure to any area by frequent position changes (every 2 hours may not be enough in high-risk patients) and range-of-motion exercises.

Other

- Teach safe use of hair-care products. Comb hair immediately when wet with large-toothed comb to prevent breakage. If scalp oils are used, encourage patient to read label for presence of irritants. Explain risks of hot-comb alopecia and irreversible damage (burns, scars) to scalp because of excessive heat.
- Pseudofolliculitis can occur from shaving curly, coarse hair. Discuss options such as growing a beard or using depilatory instead of razor.
- Sole surfaces and heels may be very calloused and cracked because of increased dry skin layers, failure to properly wash and/or clean (scraping with dull instruments or using pumice bars), improper shoe fit, and walking without shoes. Refer patient to podiatrist if unable to safely clean sole surfaces and heels or if signs of irritation or infection are observed.

- Diabetic patients should be referred to podiatrist if they have foot injuries or if they are unable to safely trim and clean toenails.
- Constricting garments (girdles, knee-high stockings, garter belts) must not be worn by patients with circulatory, endocrine, and cardiovascular problems.
- In some cultures, women do not shave body hair.

Associated Community Agencies

- Adult Protective Services (APS)
- American Academy of Dermatology
- American Cancer Society
- Skin Cancer Foundation
- National Pediculosis Association

CHAPTER **7**

Head

🔲 History

- Risk of head injury from accidents involving automobiles, cycling, sports, job, other
- Use of helmet and seat belts
- History of head injury, seizures, headaches, dizziness
- <u>Headache:</u> Location, onset, duration, character of pain, precipitating factors, associated symptoms, treatment
- Stress management techniques

- Birth trauma, difficult delivery
- Neural tube defects

(Continued on following page)

- Injuries (trauma, risk factors)
- Achieving developmental milestones

Geriatric

- Syncope, headaches, trauma
- Dizziness related to sudden movements of head or neck
- Assess for unexplained injuries to the head

Equipment

- Tape measure
- Pin or cotton ball
- Flashlight or penlight
- Stethoscope

Patient Preparation

- Sitting

Physical Assessment

Adult

Steps	Normal and/or Common Findings	Significant Deviations
Inspection		
• *Head:* Note position, movements, facial features, symmetry, shape, expressions	Upright Still	Tilted to one side; involuntary movements Tremor, bobbing, nodding Tics, spasms
	Slight asymmetry	Asymmetry: Entire side, partial, mouth only
	Uniform Appropriate	Edema, unusual shapes Flat, fixed

(Continued on following page)

(Continued)

Steps	Normal and/or Common Findings	Significant Deviations
Palpation		
• *Skull:* Note shape, symmetry	Smooth, uniform, intact	Lump, indentations
• *Temporal arteries:* Note course	Smooth, nontender	Tenderness, thickening
• *Temporomandibular joint:* Note range of motion	3–6 cm vertical range when mouth open; 1–2 cm lateral motion. snaps or pops	Pain Crepitus Inability to close or open fully
Test		
• *Cranial nerve (CN) VII:* Have patient puff cheeks, raise brows, frown, smile, show teeth	Symmetrical movement	Asymmetrical motion or absence of motion
• *CN V:* Have patient clench teeth; touch pin or cotton ball to chin, then cheek	Symmetrical movement Symmetrical response	Asymmetrical motion or absence of motion Asymmetrical or absent perception of touch
Auscultation (Only if vascular anomaly suspected; use bell only)		
• Temples, eyes, suboccipital areas, forehead		Bruits

◗ Physical Assessment

Pediatric Adaptations

INFANTS & NEWBORNS ONLY

Steps	Normal and/or Common Findings	Significant Deviations
Inspection		
• *Skull:* Note size, shape, symmetry (Fig. 7–1)	Molding* Caput succedaneum*, flat fontanels, long narrow shape if premature	Frontal bossing Cephalohematoma Dilated scalp veins Separated sutures Flattened occiput may result from prolonged supine positioning

* Newborn only

(Continued on following page)

Steps	Normal and/or Common Findings	Significant Deviations
Palpation • *Fontanels:* Note size, tension, suture lines (Hold child upright.) Posterior closes by 2 months; anterior closes between 9 and 18 months	<5 cm anterior, slight pulsation, soft fontanel	Marked pulsations or depressed fontanels; bulging, full fontanels Nonpalpable sutures Extra ridges, craniotabes
Measure • Frontal occipital circumference (FOC)	Should approximate chest circumference	Micro/macrocephaly
Transilluminate (Only if abnormality is suspected)	Light does not penetrate skull	Light glows through cranial cavity

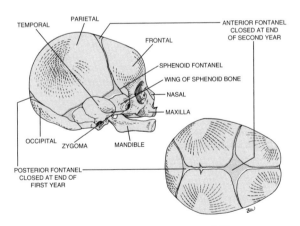

FONTANELS OF INFANT'S SKULL AND BONES OF SKULL

Figure 7-1 Fontanels of an infant's skull and bones of the skull. (*Source: Thomas, C (ed): Taber's Cyclopedic Medical Dictionary, ed 19. FA Davis, Philadelphia, 2001, p 815, with permission.*)

🔲 Physical Assessment

Pediatric Adaptations

CHILDREN

Steps	Normal and/or Common Findings	Significant Deviations
Auscultation • Eyes, temples, subocciput	Bruits common until age 4	Bruits after age 4

🔲 Physical Assessment

Geriatric Adaptations

None.

🔲 Physical Assessment

Cultural Adaptations

Steps	Normal and/or Common Findings	Significant Deviations
Inspection • Bones	Frontal bone thicker and parietal occiput not as thick in African-American males as in white males	

🔲 Diagnostic Tests

May need to refer for:
• CT scan
• MRI

Possible Nursing Diagnoses

- Trauma, risk for
- Tissue perfusion, altered, cerebral
- Injury, risk for
- Body image disturbance

 Clinical Alert

- Pediatric
  - Cephalohematoma
  - Bulging or depressed fontanels
  - Microcephaly
  - Macrocephaly
- Adult, Geriatric
  - Bruits
  - Asymmetry if marked or new
  - Hardness, thickening, or tenderness over temporal arteries, which may be associated with temporal arteritis
  - Enlarged occipital, preauricular, or postauricular lymph nodes

Sample Documentation

Face symmetrical without involuntary movements. CN V, VII intact. Skull smooth, symmetrical. Expressions appropriate to setting. Scalp without lesions or flaking. Temporal arteries without thickness or tenderness.

Patient and Family Education and Home Health Notes

Adult

- Always use helmet when cycling.
- Always use seat belts.
- Practice basic stress management techniques.
- Do not ride or carry passenger in back of pickup trucks.
- Do not drive while under the influence of alcohol or drugs.
- Do not dive into water of unknown depth.

Pediatric

- Explain various skull shapes attributable to birth procedures and indicate expected recovery time.
- Explain fontanels, including that they can be touched, and that hair should be washed.
- Strongly encourage the use of helmets when riding bicycle or skateboarding and the use of car seats and seat belts (mandatory in most states).
- Encourage parents to place infant in prone position while awake to decrease flattening of head.
- Place infant in supine or side-lying position for sleep.

Geriatric

- Provide tips related to dizziness.
- Caution patient to avoid falls. Do not use throw rugs. Use safety grips on floor of bathtub, label stairs well, and use night light in bathroom.
- Rise from lying or sitting positions to standing position slowly if dizziness occurs.
- Use cane or walker if indicated.

Other

- Patients with circulatory, endocrine, and/or cardiovascular problems should seek immediate medical attention with sudden onset of severe headaches, dizziness, blurred vision, change in level of consciousness, change in speech pattern, or irregular heart rates (high incidence and mortality rates for myocardial infarction, hypertensive crisis, and stroke).

Associated Community Agencies

- Brain Injury Association of America (formerly National Head Injury Foundation)
- Alzheimer's Association (support services, information)
- Mental Health Association

CHAPTER **8**

Neck

History

Adult

- Recent weight changes
- Changes in activity tolerance; fatigue, irritability
- Thyroid disease or surgery
- Neck stiffness, pain, and limited motion
- Temperature intolerance
- Difficulty swallowing
- Enlarged lymph nodes
- Radiation exposure
- Chemotherapy
- HIV exposure

(Continued on following page)

Adult   *(Continued)*

- IV drug use
- Recurrent infections
- Hoarseness
- Athletic injuries to neck
- Engages in heavy lifting
- Tobacco use
- Bleeding

Pediatric

Infant
- Maternal hyperthyroidism
- Quality of head control

Geriatric

- Thyroid disease, especially hypothyroidism
- Stiff neck muscles

Equipment

- Stethoscope
- Cup of water (thyroid)

Patient Preparation

- Patient should be sitting.
- Patient may need a cup of water to swallow during thyroid palpation.

Physical Assessment

Adult

Steps	Normal and/or Common Findings	Significant Deviations
Inspection		
• *Neck:* Note shape, symmetry, size	Uniform, symmetrical, proportional to head and shoulders	Masses, webbing, or fullness Unusually short Edema
• *Trachea:* Note position	Midline	Deviations to either side
• Carotid, jugular	Mild pulsations	Distention, fullness
• *Thyroid (with and without swallowing):* Note symmetry, size	Usually not visible	Marked
Palpation		
• *Trachea:* Note position, margins, motion (finger and thumb held on either side of trachea; feel for downward pull that is synchronous with pulse)	Midline, nontender, distinct rings	Edematous, deviated laterally, tender or painful, tracheal tugging
• *Thyroid:* Note size, shape, consistency, tenderness; place two fingers on each side of trachea below cricoid cartilage; feel for isthmus while patient swallows; gently push trachea to right side, have patient tilt head to left side, and feel right lobe while patient swallows; reverse and repeat; palpate lateral borders by pressing on either side of each sternocleidomastoid as patient swallows (Figs. 8–1 and 8–2)	May be nonpalpable. Right lobe may be slightly larger if palpable with swallowing	Enlarged, tender, nodules, masses, roughened surface Fixed

(Continued on following page)

(Continued)

Steps	Normal and/or Common Findings	Significant Deviations
Palpation *(Continued)* • *Lymph nodes:* Note location, mobility, size, shape, consistency, tenderness, skin margins, color (Begin with light pressure, gradually increasing to moderate pressure) see Figure 8–3 for nodes to palpate	Nonpalpable; small (≤1 cm), smooth, firm, mobile, non-tender, discrete margins	Inflamed nodes: Enlarged, tender, mobile, blurred borders, reddened skin Malignant nodes: Enlarged, nontender, fixed, hard, nodular, irregular shape, nondiscrete margins
Testing • *CN XI:* Have patient shrug shoulders with and without resistance, and have client turn head to each side against resistance	Symmetrical movement and strength	Asymmetrical or absent motion
Auscultation • *Enlarged thyroid:* Note bruits (use bell). • *Carotid arteries:* Note bruits	None None	Bruits Bruits (e.g., from aortic stenosis)

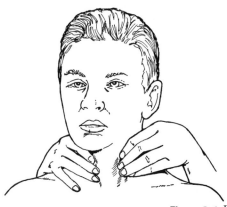

Palpating thyroid

Figure 8-1 Palpating the thyroid.

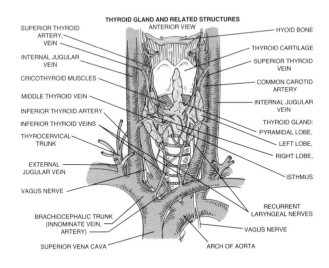

Figure 8-2 Thyroid gland and related structures. (*Source: Taber's Cyclopedic Medical Dictionary, ed 19, 2001, p 2190, with permission.*)

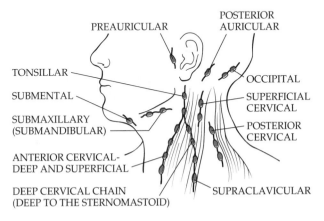

Figure 8-3 Lymph nodes of the head and neck.

◼ Physical Assessment

Pediatric Adaptations

Steps	Normal and/or Common Findings	Significant Deviations
Inspection • Assess ROM of neck; note nuchal rigidity, if any	Full ROM	Webbing Nuchal rigidity Edema Head lag past 6 months Head tilt Torticollis
Palpation • Thyroid • > 2 years: Postauricular and occipital > 1 year: Cervical, submandibular • Trachea	May not be palpable, nontender Lymph nodes may be palpable Midline, no deviations	

◼ Physical Assessment

Geriatric Adaptations

Steps	Normal and/or Common Findings	Significant Deviations
Inspection • *ROM:* Note flexibility, strength; do ROM very slowly and carefully	Decreased	Marked limitation of movement Crepitation back of neck (cervical arthritis)
Palpation • Thyroid • Lymph nodes	Small, smooth, or nonpalpable May be irregular or fibrous nodules	Pain, dizziness Enlarged lobes palpable without swallowing, tenderness
Auscultation • Carotid arteries		Bruits

Diagnostic Tests

May need to refer for:
- Infant screen, hypothyroidism
- Biopsy of enlarged lymph nodes
- Thyroid-stimulating hormone (TSH), triiodothyronine (T_3), thyroxine (T_4), (T_7)
- Carotid Doppler study

Possible Nursing Diagnoses

- Airway clearance, ineffective
- Activity intolerance, risk for
- Swallowing, impaired
- Aspiration, risk for

Clinical Alert

- Obstructed airway
- Palpable supraclavicular nodes, always refer
- Suspicious nodes, refer
- Enlarged, nodular thyroid, refer
- Hypothyroidism frequently not diagnosed in older patients and assumed to be depression. Monitor for symptoms such as fatigue, activity intolerance, constipation, decreased appetite, dry skin, or mood changes.

Sample Documentation

Neck smooth, supple, with full ROM. Trachea aligned in midline. No jugular venous distention. Thyroid not visible, not palpable. No tenderness. CN XI intact. Lymph nodes (auricular, occipital, clavicular, cervical, tonsillar, submaxillary, submental) not palpable. No carotid bruits bilaterally.

Patient and Family Education and Home Health Notes

Adult

- Self-referral of enlarged suspicious nodes, difficulty swallowing

Pediatric

- <u>Infants:</u> Thoroughly clean skin folds in neck.
- <u>Infants:</u> No pillows or soft stuffed animals should be allowed in crib. Mattress should be firm.
- Never shake infant or child (significant risk for injury of head or neck).

Geriatric

- Refer patient for thyroid tests if he or she reports low energy.
- Exercise neck muscles to maintain as much mobility as possible (flexion, extension. hyperextension, rotation, and lateral flexion).
- If several pillows are used, place part of pillows under shoulder to prevent prolonged extreme neck flexion.

CHAPTER 9

Eyes

🞄 History

Adult

- Date and source of last eye exam: age at time of exam
- Use of corrective lenses; if so, type, how long
- History (self or family) of hypertension, diabetes, allergies, thyroid disorder, glaucoma, medications, color blindness
- History of previous eye surgery, trauma, infection
- <u>Employment</u>: Risk of Injury
- Participation in athletic activities, use of protective devices
- Headache
- Pain, burning, itching, drying, tearing, discharge
- Blurred vision
- Lights, spots, floaters
- Recent changes in vision
- Allergies

Pediatric

- <u>Preterm</u>: Resuscitated, oxygen therapy
- Maternal rubella while pregnant
- Ability to follow object and fixate with eyes
- Squinting to see objects; rubbing of eyes
- Age, date, and source of last eye exam; age at time of exam
- Headaches when reading
- Reversals of written numbers and/or letters
- Trouble reading correctly
- Sitting close to the television at home
- Excessive tearing
- Retinal hemorrhages in young child

(Continued on following page)

- History of glaucoma, diabetes, cataracts, or macular degeneration (wet or dry)
- Decreased vision, difficulty reading or seeing at night
- Peripheral or central vision blurred
- History of glaucoma in family; any acute eye pain
- Long, excessive exposure to sunlight
- Bothered by glaring lights
- Bothered by rainbows around lights or halos around lights
- Difficulty distinguishing colors
- Dry eyes
- Increased eye tearing
- Double vision, tunnel vision, or transient blindness
- Use of corrective lenses; used for what purpose?
- Use of any aids (magnifier) or any environmental adaptations to see better
- History of floaters (spots) and flashes of light

Other

- Retinoblastoma, cancer of retina
- History of strabismus
- Nocturnal eye pain

▨ Equipment

- Penlight
- Rosenbaum Pocket Vision Screener chart (Fig. 9–1) or newsprint
- Snellen Tumbling E chart*
- Ophthalmoscope
- Clean cotton wisp
- Cover card

* Use Snellen Tumbling E chart (see Fig. 9–7) for children 3–7 years old.

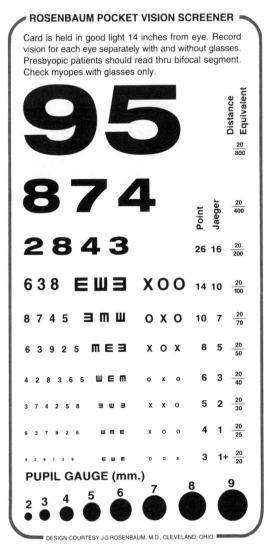

Figure 9-1 Rosenbaum pocket vision screener. (*Source: Dr. J. George Rosenbaum, FACS, Cleveland, Ohio, with permission.*)

🔖 Patient Preparation

- Patient should be in a sitting position.
- Explain darkening of room for ophthalmic exam.
- Explain use of cotton to elicit blink.

🔖 Physical Assessment: External Eyes

Adult

Steps	Normal and/or Common Findings	Significant Deviations
Inspection		
• *Bony orbit, brows, lacrimal apparatus, eye:* Note symmetry, size, position (Fig. 9–2)	Equal size and movement	Exophthalmos Strabismus
• *Lids:* Note position, motion, symmetry, lesions	Symmetrical blink; lashes even and curl out, moist Xanthelasma	Edema, ptosis, exudate, ectropion, hordeolum
• *Iris:* Note color, shape	Uniform color, round	Coloboma, iridectomy
• *Cornea, lens (with oblique light)*	Clear, smooth, moist	Opaque, arcus senilis before age 40
• Note cloudiness of lens		Cataract
• *Pupil:* Note shape, symmetry, response to light	PERRLA: Pupils equal, round, reactive to light and accommodation Consensual	Not equal in shape; response to light unequal, slow, absent, diminished

(Continued on following page)

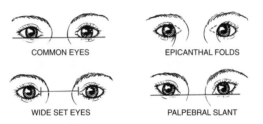

Figure 9-2 Placement of eyes.

Steps	Normal and/or Common Findings	Significant Deviations
• *Pupil:* Note accommodation; focus distant object, then close (Fig. 9–3)	Constricts for close object, convergence present	Miosis, mydriasis Fails to respond to focus change
• *Conjunctivae:* Note color, continuity, vascularity	Clear with multiple small vessels	Reddened, exudate, lesions, jaundice
Palpation		
• Bony orbit	Firm, nontender	Tenderness
• Lacrimal apparatus	Pink, moist puncta	Tenderness, drainage, reddened, edema
Testing Eye Function		
• *CN II:* Rosenbaum Pocket Vision Screener chart at 14 in (see Fig. 9–1); have patient cover one eye, test uncovered eye; test with lenses if patient already uses glasses or contacts; test OD, OS, OU	20/20 without straining *Near vision:* Reads at 14 in	Decreased acuity, e.g., 20/40 Moves closer or farther than 14 in for reading
• *Confrontation test:* With your eyes level with patient's eyes, stand 2 ft from patient and cover one eye while patient covers opposite eye; look at each other; move object into superior, inferior, nasal, and temporal fields for each eye (Fig. 9–4)	Object seen by both at same time	Diminished peripheral vision

(Continued on page 133)

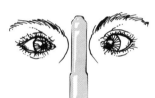

Figure 9-3 Checking for optical accommodation and convergence.

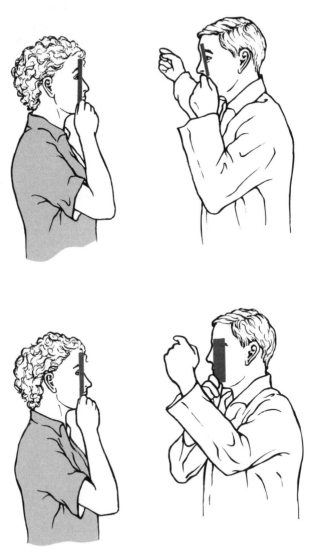

Figure 9-4 Testing peripheral fields of vision.

(Continued)

Steps	Normal and/or Common Findings	Significant Deviations
Testing Eye Function *(Continued)*		
• *CN III, IV, VI, and extraocular muscles:* Hold patient's chin, have patient focus eyes on pencil held at comfortable distance from eyes; instruct patient to follow pencil with eyes as pencil is moved through six cardinal fields of gaze (Fig. 9–5)	Smooth, equal movements	Nystagmus Lid lag
• Shine light obliquely into each pupil	Equal pupillary constriction	Asymmetry or absence of pupillary constriction
• Muscle balance with corneal light reflex; shine light on corneas while patient looks straight ahead	Symmetrical reflection of light	Asymmetry; strabismus, hypertelorism
• *CN V:* Touch wisp of cotton to cornea to elicit blink reflex (alert patient before touching with cotton)	Blink symmetrical and complete	Asymmetrical, incomplete, or absent blink response

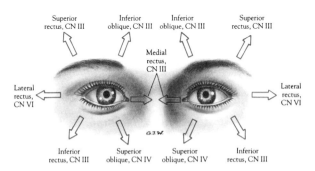

Figure 9-5 Extraocular eye muscles (EOM). (*Source: Seidel, H, Ball, J, Dains, J, and Benedict, GW: Mosby's Physical Examination Handbook, ed 3. Mosby, St. Louis, 2003, p 67, with permission.*)

Physical Assessment: Internal Eyes

Adult

Darken room. Have patient focus on object over your shoulder. OD: ophthalmoscope in right hand, focus with numbered wheel. OS: ophthalmoscope in left hand. (Procedure is tiring for patient.)

Steps	Normal and/or Common Findings	Significant Deviations
Inspection		
• Red reflex	Present Round, reddish orange	Cataract; hemorrhage may appear solid or as dots
• *Retina:* Note color	Yellowish pink, uniform	Marked dark colors, lesions, folds in retina
• *Disk:* Note color, size, shape, margins of disk, and cup	Yellow to pink, round, 1.5 mm, sharply defined border, cup 40%–50% of disk, lighter color in center of disk	Papilledema, cupping with white color, vessels visible in disk
• *Vessels:* Note color, size, junctions	Size A3:V5, arterioles bright red	Cup less or more than 40%–50% of disk
• *Macula densa and fovea centralis:* Note location, color (Fig. 9–6); difficult to locate unless pupils are dilated	Located two disk diameters temporal to disk, bright yellow	Arteriovenous (AV) nicking, areas of constriction

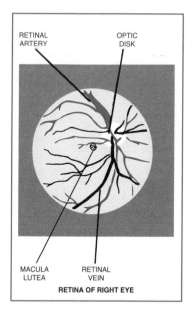

Figure 9-6 Retina of right eye. (*Source: Taber's Cyclopedic Medical Dictionary, ed 19, 2001, p 1874, with permission.*)

Physical Assessment: External and Internal Eyes

Pediatric Adaptations

INFANT AND CHILD

Steps	Normal and/or Common Findings	Significant Deviations
Inspection • *External eye:* Note spacing, symmetry (see Fig. 9–2)	Symmetrically positioned and spaced	Sunken eyes Edema of lids, epicanthal folds (abnormal except in Asians), hypertelorism

(Continued on following page)

(Continued)

Steps	Normal and/or Common Findings	Significant Deviations
Inspection (continued)		
• Ability of infant to gaze at parent and blink appropriately		Failure to gaze and blink Setting sun sign
• *Conjunctivae:* Note color, clarity	Pink, moist	Drainage Excessive tearing Pallor
• Muscle balance	Symmetrical movement, pseudostrabismus	Strabismus, nystagmus
• Red reflex	Present	Cataract
Child Testing		
• Visual acuity (Snellen Tumbling E chart [Fig. 9–7] for ages 3–7; not accurate < age 3)	Age 1:20/200 Age 2: 20/70 Age 5: 20/30 Age 6: 20/20	Two-line difference between eyes 4-year-old with acuity of 20/40 or less
• Color differentiation check at age 5	Differentiates colors	Color blindness

◼ Physical Assessment: External and Internal Eyes

Geriatric Adaptations

Steps	Normal and/or Common Findings	Significant Deviations
Inspection		
• *Lids:* Note position		Lid lag, ptosis, ectropion, entropion
• Sclera: note color		Senile hyaline Plaque Arcus senilis
• *Pupils:* Note size	Diminished	

(Continued on page 138)

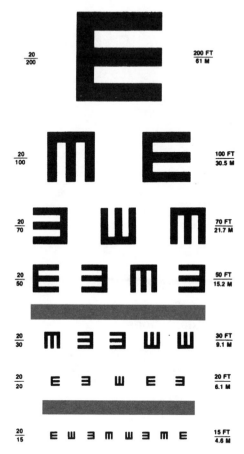

Figure 9-7 The Snellen Tumbling E chart. (***Source:*** *Adapted from Vision Screening Manual, Texas Department of Health, Austin, TX, 1998, p 22, used with permission.*)

(Continued)

Steps	Normal and/or Common Findings	Significant Deviations
Inspection (continued)		
• *Cornea:* Note clarity	Arcus senilis Diminished visual acuity Diminished adaptation to dark	Cloudy or opaque, abrasions, ulcerations
• *Lens:* Note clarity. *Test each eye separately*	Clear	Cloudiness, opacity
Geriatric Testing		
• *Visual acuity/Snellen chart:* Use lightened chart or a light behind the patient. Test with and without corrective lenses	20/20 to 20/30 with corrective lenses	Any line above the 20/30 line on the chart

Physical Assessment: External and Internal Eyes

Cultural Adaptations

Steps	Normal and/or Common Findings	Significant Deviations
Inspection		
• *Sclera:* Note color	Slight yellow cast Brown spots	Dots of pigmentation near corneal limbus
• *Eyeball:* Note position	May protrude slightly beyond supraorbital ridge	
• Fundi (A-A)	Heavily pigmented; uniformly dark	
• Conjunctivae		Pale
• Internal eye		Detached retina (severe sickle cell)

Diagnostic Tests

May need to refer for:

- Mydriatic agent to dilate pupils for full fundoscopic exam
- Puff test for pressure in glaucoma

Possible Nursing Diagnoses

- Sensory-perceptual alterations, visual
- Social interaction, impaired
- Social isolation

Clinical Alert

- Explain possible discomfort of light and cotton wisp.
- Do not use light in eyes for excessively long times.
- If red reflex is absent, reposition scope.
- If patient experiences sudden eye pain, large flashes of light, loss of vision, discharge, redness, or swelling, refer to an ophthalmologist as soon as possible.

Sample Documentation

Eyes: Symmetrical with no lag or turning of lids; no exophthalmos noted. Sclera clear, white; conjunctivae dark pink without inflammation. Irises light blue, intact. PERRLA. Extraocular muscles (EOMs) and normal visual fields intact (CN III, IV, VI). Alignment and convergence normal. Corneal reflex intact (CN V). Fundoscopic: Disks flat, yellow. No AV nicking, hemorrhage, or cupping noted; A3:V5. Acuity (CN II): OD 20/40, OS 20/20, OU 20/20. Corrected (Rosenbaum chart).

■ Patient and Family Education and Home Health notes

General

- Use wraparound sunglasses with UV protection when outdoors.

Adult

- Recommend examination every 5 to 10 years until age 40, then every 2 to 5 years.
- Stress use of safety glasses with hobbies, home repair.

Pediatric

Infants
- Explain normal vision: (i.e., poor acuity and poor muscle control at birth, lack of tears until 3 months).

Children and Adolescents
- Use sunglasses when outdoors, especially when in the sun or in highly reflective area (e.g., sand, water, snow).
- Vision should be screened at ages 3, 4 to 6, 7 to 9, and 13.
- Color vision should be screened at 4 to 5 years of age.
- Use protective eyewear when performing hazardous activities.

Geriatric

- Explain drying of mucous membranes, possible need for artificial lubricants.
- Recommend examination every year and as necessary when changes occur.
- Emphasize that blindness caused by glaucoma or cataracts is preventable or treatable if detected early and that eye drops for glaucoma must be taken for a lifetime.

(Continued on following page)

- Inform patient of visual side effects of any medications being taken.
- Use bright, indirect lighting when performing fine tasks (reading, sewing).
- Use a magnifier for fine tasks if necessary.
- Inform patient of the availability of large-print books and reading materials.
- <u>Symptoms that require immediate attention:</u> Pain, discharge, redness or swelling, loss of vision, excessive tearing, floaters that occur in association with light flashes.

Cultural ▶

- Encourage testing for glaucoma every 1 to 2 years in African-Americans because of their high risk.
- Certain cultural groups may respond differently to treatments (Jarvis, 2000).

Associated Community Agencies

- American Society for the Blind: Talking books, adaptive aids for the home
- Foundation for Glaucoma Research: Education and support
- Lion's Club: May provide glasses for children or adults
- Local optometry schools: Discounted eye exams
- National Society to Prevent Blindness: Information and local services such as eye exams
- National Association for Parents of the Visually Impaired: Provides support and promotes public understanding

CHAPTER **10**

Ears

🔲 History

- Changes in hearing acuity, changes in speech sounds
- Aids to hearing used
- Vertigo, dizziness, earaches, drainage
- Exposure to loud sounds in the past
- Medications affecting hearing, especially antibiotics
- Methods of hygiene
- History of renal disease, diabetes in self or family
- History of sinusitis, streptococcal infections
- History of Ménière's disease
- History of ear surgery, trauma

Infants
- Prematurity
- Maternal syphilis, rubella
- Exposure to antibiotics
- Chronic otitis media or upper respiratory infections
- Exposure to passive smoke
- Pulling or tugging at ears
- No increasing pattern of prespeech sounds/speech
- No reaction to loud noise
- Foul odor
- Allergies

(Continued on following page)

Adolescents
- <u>Exposure to loud noises:</u> Chronic, acute, amount
- Frequency and sites of swimming
- Protrusion of external ear

- Hearing ringing or crackling noises
- Conversations of others sounding garbled or distorted
- Use of a hearing aid and its effectiveness
- Recurrent problems with cerumen impactions
- Frequently asking others to repeat themselves or keeping volume of radio or television turned up high
- Earache, dizziness, vertigo
- Hearing loss accompanied by suspiciousness, depression, social withdrawal, confusion
- Time of last audiometric examination
- Long-term exposure to loud noise

Equipment

- Otoscope
- Tuning fork
- Ticking watch
- Audiometer (if appropriate to setting)

Patient Preparation

- Patient should be sitting.
- Tip head away from ear being examined.
- Parent may hold infant or toddler against parent's chest for otoscope exam.

Physical Assessment: External Ear

Adult

Steps	Normal and/or Common Findings	Significant Deviations
Inspection		
• Position of ear in relation to eye (Fig. 10–1)	Ear should be nearly upright, angling <10° toward occiput.	Unequal alignment, pinna below line level with corner of eye
• *Auricles:* Note size, shape, color, symmetry	Color of skin, uniform shape	Masses, lesions, deformities, cyanosis, erythema, edema
Palpation		
• Ear lobes	Smooth, uniform edge	Tophi, nodules
• Tragus, helix	Nontender	Tenderness, pain, ulcers
• Mastoid	Nontender	Edema, tenderness, masses
Testing Hearing Function: Test CN VIII		
• *Weber:* Place vibrating fork at midsagittal line (Fig. 10-2)	Patient should hear or sense vibrations equally in both ears	*Sound lateralized to one ear:* Perceptive loss from nerve damage, goes to unaffected ear Conductive loss from otosclerosis, goes to affected ear
• *Rinne:* Place vibrating fork on mastoid. After vibrations are no longer felt, hold fork beside ear to hear (see Fig. 10-2)	Air conduction = 2 × bone conduction; able to hear vibrations after feeling stops (air conduction greater than bone conduction)	If air conduction >2 × bone conduction, there is perceptive loss. If air conduction <2 × bone conduction, there is conductive loss
• Whisper test: Occlude one of patient's ears and whisper 1-2 ft lateral to opposite ear	Patient should be able to hear half of all words whispered	Unable to hear
• Watch test. Start at about 18 in away from ear and compare with a person with normal hearing	Able to hear at approximately the same distance as others with normal hearing are able to hear the same watch	Unable to hear

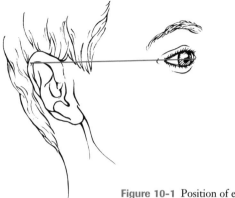

Figure 10-1 Position of eye and ear.

🔲 Physical Assessment: Canal, Membrane

Adult

Steps	Normal and/or Common Findings	Significant Deviations
Inspection		
• Anchor otoscope on patient's head, tilted away from you; pull auricle up, out, and back to straighten auditory canal and *gently* insert speculum to depth of approximately 1/2 in (Fig. 10-3)		
• *Canal:* Note appearance of canal color; amount, type, and site of cerumen	Moist brown cerumen, cilia	Foreign bodies, discharge, lesions, foul odor, edema, flaking, erythema, moderate to severe pain on insertion
• *Tympanic membrane:* Note landmarks (umbo, cone of light, malleus handles), color (Fig. 10-4), integrity	Silver-gray color, shiny, conical, intact; old scars appear as white marks; cone of light at 5 o'clock position in right ear and at 7 o'clock position in left ear	Bulging (unable to note landmarks) or retracting (pronounced landmarks) Perforations, foul odor, discharge Dull, red, blue

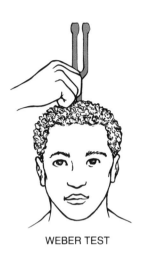

WEBER TEST

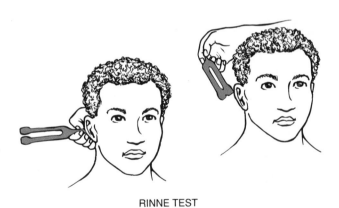

RINNE TEST

Figure 10-2 Weber test and Rinne test.

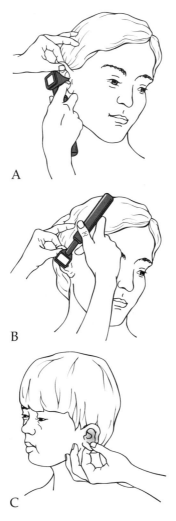

Figure 10-3 Use of otoscope. (*A, B*) Adult. (*C*) Child.

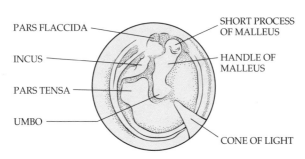

Figure 10-4 The tympanic membrane and landmarks of right ear.

▰ Physical Assessment: External Ear, Canal, Membrane

Pediatric Adaptations

INFANT

Steps	Normal and/or Common Findings	Significant Deviations
Inspection		
• *External:* Note shape and placement; draw an imaginary line from the inner canthus of the eye to the outer canthus of the eye	Uniform size and shape Recoils briskly Top of ear intersects this line	Preauricular pits, dimples, skin tags Unusual shapes Low-set ears Slow or absent recoil Foul odor
• *Canal:* Stabilize head, restrain child firmly if needed, gently pull auricle down and back	Vernix in canal (newborn)	Foreign body
• *Tympanic membrane:* Use pneumatic otoscope to differentiate from illness	If membrane is red, may be caused by crying	Fluid, edema, bulging, marked reddening Loss of bony landmarks Nonmobile tympanic membrane

(Continued on following page)

Steps	Normal and/or Common Findings	Significant Deviations
Test • Infant • 4–6 months old • 8–10 months old • 12 months old • *3–4 years old:* Use Weber or Rinne test	Flattened startle (Moro) or blink reflex Turns to sounds Responds to name Begins to imitate words	Delayed or absent response

🔲 Physical Assessment: External Ear, Canal, Membrane

Geriatric Adaptations

Steps	Normal and/or Common Findings	Significant Deviations
Inspection • *Auricles:* Note size • *Cerumen:* Note amount, consistency, color	Women may have large sagging lobes if they have worn heavy earrings for many years	 Dry, dark, impacted cerumen

🔲 Physical Assessment: External Ear, Canal, Membrane

Cultural Adaptations

Steps	Normal and/or Common Findings	Significant Deviations
Inspection • *Cerumen:* Note consistency, color	Dry, light brown to gray color in Asians, Native Americans	

🔲 Diagnostic Tests

May need to refer to:
* Audiometric testing

🔲 Possible Nursing Diagnoses

* Communication, impaired verbal
* Social isolation
* Self-esteem disturbance
* Injury, risk for

 Clinical Alert

* Refer to otolaryngologist for severe tenderness, pain, lesions, discharge, foreign bodies, and/or progressive hearing loss or ringing in the ears.

🔲 Sample Documentation

Verbal and nonverbal communication congruent and appropriate to setting. Auricles in alignment. Pinnae pink, elastic, symmetrical, without lesions, deformities, or tenderness. Auditory canals unobstructed, moderate amount of dark brown, moist cerumen present; tympanic membrane visualized intact, shiny and gray bilaterally; bony landmarks and light reflex present; no bulging, retractions, or redness. Vibratory sense intact; CN VIII intact with whisper test.

Patient and Family Education and Home Health Notes

Adult

- Do not attempt to clean or remove wax with a cotton swab or other device.
- Use washcloth or finger in outer ear.
- If canal needs cleaning, irrigate with bulb syringe, soaking with oil if necessary.
- Avoid excessively loud sounds or use ear plugs.

Pediatric

- Ear infections are common and potentially dangerous. Do not put to bed with bottles of milk or other fluids. Be aware that colds and mild upper respiratory infections may develop into ear infections.
- Explain increased risk of otitis media for infants through preschoolers.
- Clean only outer ear using damp cloth.
- Child may insert objects into ears. Take child to healthcare provider for removal of all objects.
- Eliminate exposure to smoke.
- Audiometric testing should be given to preschooler.
- Caution about loud music, especially when played through headphones.

Geriatric

- Have hearing tested annually by a physician or audiologist.
- Obtain a variety of hearing devices for the home, such as telephones with louder ringing mechanism and earpiece amplification, louder door chimes, wireless infrared TV listener.
- Do not be afraid to tell people to face you, speak at a slightly slower rate, use lower voice tones, be very clear, and to not shout.

(Continued on following page)

- Teach how to care for hearing aids; explain that hearing aids should not be purchased unless recommended by a physician or audiologist. Purchase only from a reputable company (check with the Better Business Bureau).
  - Remove the hearing aid before going to bed, bathing, or showering.
  - Make sure the battery is inserted correctly. If there is no on-off switch, open the battery case at night to conserve the battery.
  - Clean the ear mold daily with a damp cloth. Once a week, wipe the mold with a cloth dampened with mild, soapy water. If the hearing aid ear mold gets plugged with ear wax, *carefully* remove the wax with a toothpick or bent paperclip.
  - Change the batteries every 10 days to 2 weeks. A whistle should be heard when the volume control is fully on.
  - Remember, the aid makes sounds and voices louder, not clearer. Expectations should be realistic.
  - Background noises may be annoying at first. Patients will most likely get used to the extraneous noise in a short time. Background noises can be turned off or down with some new hearing aids.
  - If you are having any problems with the aid, have the aid tested by a reputable audiologist or hearing aid dealer.

■ Associated Community Agencies

- American Speech-Language-Hearing Association: Education, Helpline
- American Tinnitus Association: Self-help groups
- Better Hearing Institute: Hearing Helpline
- National Association of the Deaf: Information
- National Information Center on Deafness: Information on assistive devices
- Self-Help for Hard of Hearing People, Inc.: Information and support
- American Society for Deaf Children

CHAPTER **11**

Nose and Sinuses

 History

Adult

- Stuffiness, discharge: character, onset, duration, treatment
- Seasonality of symptoms
- Sore throat
- Infections
- Epistaxis: Cause, duration, treatment, associated symptoms
- Allergies: use of nose drops and/or sprays, antihistamines, decongestants
- Repeated sinus infections
- Changes in appetite, smell sense
- Cocaine use
- History of surgery and/or trauma
- Snoring, daytime sleepiness
- Chronic alcohol abuse

Pediatric

- Nasal quality of voice
- Horizontal nasal crease ("allergic salute")
- Rhinitis
- Playing with small objects near nose

Geriatric

- Constant drainage from nose to throat
- Allergies, sneezing
- Pain

🔲 Equipment

- Penlight
- Nasal speculum

🔲 Patient Preparation

- Sitting

🔲 Physical Assessment: External

Adult

Steps	Normal and/or Common Findings	Significant Deviations
Inspection • *Nose:* Note shape, symmetry, color, discharge	Varies Uniform, symmetrical, scant	Bullous, flaring, discharge (watery, purulent, mucoid, bloody), mucus, crusting
Palpation • *Nose:* Note masses, tenderness	Straight, nontender	Masses, tenderness
• *Patency:* With patient's mouth closed, occlude each naris to assess patency of opposite side	Patent	Occluded
• *Frontal sinuses:* Press upward with thumbs under brow ridge	Nontender	Tenderness, pain
• *Maxillary sinuses:* Press up with thumbs under zygomatic arch; press in over maxillary sinus	Nontender	Tenderness, pain

(Continued on following page)

Steps	Normal and/or Common Findings	Significant Deviations
Test		
• *CN I:* Test each naris separately for ability to perceive and identify odors.	Distinguishes odors	Unable to distinguish odors
• Use a different scent for each naris		
Percussion		
• Frontal and maxillary sinuses	Nontender	Tenderness, edema

🔲 Physical Assessment: Internal

Adult

Steps	Normal and/or Common Findings	Significant Deviations
Inspection		
• Tilt head back to insert speculum 1 cm. Avoid touching septum with speculum		
• *Nares:* Note color, mucosa	Pink and moist	Masses, lesions, redness, foreign bodies
		Polyps, fissures, ulcers, discharge, bleeding
• *Inferior, middle, and superior turbinates:* Note color, consistency	Pink, smooth (same-color as mucosa)	Redness, pallor, edema
• *Septum:* Note integrity, alignment	Straight Uniform	Deviation attributable to trauma, bleeding

Pediatric Adaptations

INFANT

Steps	Normal and/or Common Findings	Significant Deviations
Inspection • *Nose:* Note shape of bridge	Straight	

CHILD

Steps	Normal and/or Common Findings	Significant Deviations
Inspection • *Nose:* Note horizontal crease: note if mouth or nose breather	No crease Breathes through nose	Flaring horizontal crease possible sign of allergies Consistently breathes through mouth; clearly audible breath sounds
Palpation • Sphenoid, maxillary, ethmoid sinus (preschool child) • Frontal sinus (7–8 years of age)	Nontender Nontender	Tender Tender

■ Physical Assessment: nose and Sinuses

Geriatric Adaptations

Steps	Normal and/or Common Findings	Significant Deviations
Inspection • *Nose:* Note size	Appears larger and more prominent with age	
Test • Sense of smell	Diminishes with age	Absent

Physical Assessment: Nose and Sinuses

Cultural Adaptations

Steps	Normal and/or Common Findings	Significant Deviations
Inspection • *Nose:* Note shape, size	Size and shape vary in different cultural groups	

Diagnostic Tests

May need to refer for
• Biopsy of suspicious lesions

Possible Nursing Diagnoses

• Breathing pattern, ineffective
• Injury, risk for
• Airway clearance, ineffective
• Aspiration, risk for
• Communication, impaired verbal

Clinical Alert

• Prevent trauma to nasal mucosa with use of nasal speculum, nasal catheter, or nasogastric feeding tube.

🔖 Sample Documentation

Nose aligned, symmetrical, without discharge or redness. Both nares patent, no tenderness or masses palpated. Mucosa and septum without redness, swelling, or lesions. Sinuses not tender. CN I intact; distinguishes aromas correctly.

🔖 Patient and Family Education and Home Health Notes

Adult

- Prevent trauma to sensitive mucous membranes of nose.

Pediatric

- Avoid insertion of foreign bodies into nose. If object has been inserted, take child to physician's office for removal if foreign body is not easily grasped.
- Demonstrate use of tissue and handwashing to prevent spread of upper respiratory infection (URI).

Geriatric

- If sense of smell is diminished, teach patient to routinely check and turn off dials on gas stoves (to prevent asphyxiation) and to label with a specific date foods stored in the refrigerator (to prevent eating spoiled foods).
- Inspect pilot lights periodically to lessen risk of gas exposure.
- Have smoke detector installed in home and test every 6 months. Need detector that flashes light if person has major hearing deficit.

CHAPTER **12**

Mouth and Throat

History

Adult

- <u>Oral hygiene practices:</u> Method, products used, frequency
- <u>Dental apparatus:</u> Braces, dentures, bridges, or crowns
- Date of last dental exam
- Nutritional habits
- <u>Tobacco use:</u> Type, frequency, duration
- <u>Alcohol use:</u> Frequency, duration
- Pain
- Lesions
- Sore throat
- Hoarseness, change in voice
- Cough
- Difficulty chewing or swallowing
- History of herpes simplex, diabetes mellitus, periodontal disease, frequent streptococcal infections, tonsillectomy
- Medications that cause gum inflammation (e.g., dilantin)
- <u>Medications that diminish salivation:</u> Diuretics, antihistamines, anticholinergics, antihypertensives, antispasmodics, antidepressants

Pediatric

- Congenital defect
- Dental hygiene
- Number of teeth present
- Fluoridated water
- Use of bottle and/or pacifier
- Thumb sucking
- Sore throats

(Continued on following page)

Geriatric

- Date of last dental exam
- Soreness or bleeding lips, gums, tongue, or throat
- Missing teeth or difficulty chewing
- If appropriate, state of repair and fit of dentures
- Dry mouth
- Alterations in taste
- Oral hygiene habits
- If dentures are used, note wearing habits, how old they are, how well they fit, and if they are in good repair.
- Assess for alteration in taste that may be related to antihypertensives and certain cardiac medications. Check if the patient has a mechanical heart valve because antibiotics are needed before any dental procedures.
- History of aspiration pneumonia. Symptoms of swallowing problems, such as frequent coughing and/or choking with eating and drinking, or drooling; delayed coughing noted after finished eating or drinking.

Equipment

- Light
- Gloves (clean)
- Gauze square
- Tongue depressor

Patient Preparation

- Sitting

▧ Physical Assessment: Mouth and Tongue

Adult

Steps	Normal and/or Common Findings	Significant Deviations
Inspection		
• *Lips:* Note color, symmetry, continuity at squamous-buccal junction (Fig. 12–1)	Pink, slight asymmetry, intact	Lesions, involuntary movement, cracks, fissures, drooping, cyanosis
• *Mucosa and gums:* Note color, integrity, adherence	Pink, intact, moist	Redness, edema, lesions, masses, bleeding, cyanosis
• *Stensen's and Wharton's ducts:* Note color	Smooth, pink	Redness, edema
• *Teeth:* Note number, color, hygiene	Complete, white, clean	Multiple caries, missing teeth, fuzzy, dirty
• *Tongue:* Note size; check lateral, dorsal, and ventral surfaces for color, coating, texture, vessels	Fits comfortably in mouth with teeth together. Pink to red with papillae present. Midline fissures present. Geographic tongue	Coated, white patches, pale, nodules, ulcers. Papillae or fissures absent
• *Palate, oropharynx, uvula:* Note color, continuity, integrity	Pink; hard palate firm with rugae, soft palate spongy, uvula in midline	Redness, edema, lesions, pigmented lesions. Uvula deviated: Note direction. Softened hard palate
• *Tonsils:* Note color, size, discharge	Pink to red 1+ to 2+	Exudate 3+ to 4+. Markedly reddened

(Continued on following page)

(Continued)

Steps	Normal and/or Common Findings	Significant Deviations
Test • *CN XII:* Have patient extend tongue and move side to side	Tongue centrally aligned without fasciculations	No central alignment, fasciculations
• *CN IX, X:* Observe soft palate and uvula rising as patient says "ah"; after alerting patient, gently touch back of tongue with tongue depressor to elicit gag reflex	Soft palate rising symmetrically, uvula in midline, quick gag reflex	Unequal or absent rise of soft palate; uvula deviated on rising Absent or diminished gag reflex
Palpate (Wearing gloves) • Check lips • Assess gums	Soft, smooth	Inflammation, edema, swelling, bleeding, receding from teeth Induration, lesions
• *Tongue:* Ask patient to protrude tongue; grasp tip with gauze square and gently pull to each side; palpate sides of tongue	Muscular Nontender, smooth Pink, moist, slightly rough Midline position Voluntary movement Symmetry of shape	Tender, masses, redness Fasciculations Tumors
• Check teeth	*Position and/or condition:* Stable, smooth	Loose, broken, irregular edges
Smell • Assess oral cavity	No odor, tobacco, smoke, food odors	Foul, acetone, alcohol odor

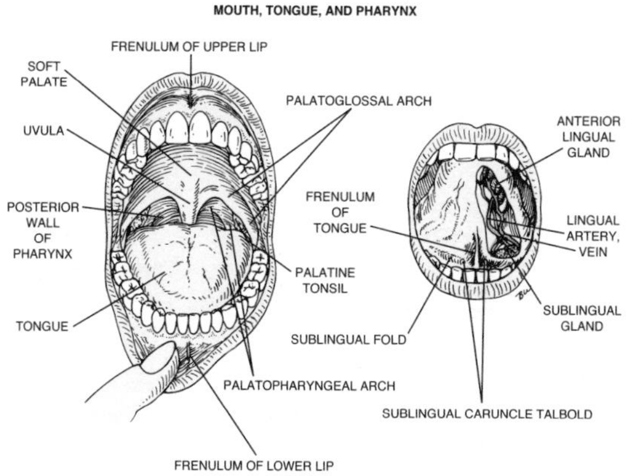

MOUTH, TONGUE, AND PHARYNX

Figure 12-1 Mouth, tongue, and pharynx. (***Source:*** *Taber's Cyclopedic Medical, Dictionary, 2001, ed 19, p 1381, with permission.*)

Physical Assessment: Mouth and Tongue

Pediatric Adaptations

INFANT

Steps	Normal and/or Common Findings	Significant Deviations
Inspection		
• Assess oral cavity	Pink Epstein's pearls, retention cysts	Thrush
• *Buccal mucosa:* Note amount and thickness of saliva, integrity of tissue	Midline uvula, freely movable Small tonsils	Cyanosis Cleft palate, lip, or bifid uvula Excessive drooling in newborn
• *Deciduous teeth:* Note number, development, eruption dates (Fig. 12-2)		
• *Tongue:* Note size	Fits in mouth with teeth closed	Large, protruding Ankyloglossia
Palpate		
• Observe soft and hard palate	Intact	Clefts

■ Physical Assessment: Mouth and Tongue

Pediatric Adaptations

CHILD

Steps	Normal and/or Common Findings	Significant Deviations
Inspection • *Arch of palate:* Note color • *Teeth:* Note number, color • *Tonsils:* Note size	Koplik's spots Malocclusion at age 8 Hypertrophic in mid-childhood	 No teeth by age 1 Inflamed, red, edematous

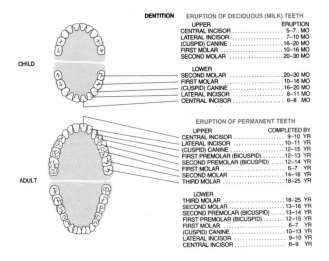

DENTITION

ERUPTION OF DECIDUOUS (MILK) TEETH

UPPER	ERUPTION
CENTRAL INCISOR	5–7 MO
LATERAL INCISOR	7–10 MO
(CUSPID) CANINE	16–20 MO
FIRST MOLAR	10–16 MO
SECOND MOLAR	20–30 MO

LOWER	
SECOND MOLAR	20–30 MO
FIRST MOLAR	10–16 MO
(CUSPID) CANINE	16–20 MO
LATERAL INCISOR	8–11 MO
CENTRAL INCISOR	6–8 MO

ERUPTION OF PERMANENT TEETH

UPPER	COMPLETED BY
CENTRAL INCISOR	9–10 YR
LATERAL INCISOR	10–11 YR
(CUSPID) CANINE	12–15 YR
FIRST PREMOLAR (BICUSPID)	12–13 YR
SECOND PREMOLAR (BICUSPID)	12–14 YR
FIRST MOLAR	6–7 YR
SECOND MOLAR	14–16 YR
THIRD MOLAR	18–25 YR

LOWER	
THIRD MOLAR	18–25 YR
SECOND MOLAR	13–16 YR
SECOND PREMOLAR (BICUSPID)	13–14 YR
FIRST PREMOLAR (BICUSPID)	12–15 YR
FIRST MOLAR	6–7 YR
(CUSPID) CANINE	10–13 YR
LATERAL INCISOR	9–10 YR
CENTRAL INCISOR	8–9 YR

CHILD

ADULT

Figure 12-2 Dentition (eruption of teeth). (*Source: Taber's Cyclopedic Medical, Dictionary, 2001, ed 19, p 557, with permission.*)

Physical Assessment: Mouth and Tongue

Pediatric Adaptations

ADOLESCENT

Steps	Normal and/or Common Findings	Significant Deviations
Inspection • *Teeth:* Note presence of 2nd and 3rd molars (see Fig. 12–2)		

Physical Assessment: Mouth and Tongue

Geriatric Adaptations

Steps	Normal and/or Common Findings	Significant Deviations
Inspection • Lips	Smaller, decreased fat pad	Leukoplakia, lesions, cracks in corners
• Teeth	Darkened, worn down	Multiple obvious caries, missing teeth
• *Gums:* Ask patient to remove dentures to see gums	May be atrophied	Irritation, lesions, bleeding, inflammation, swelling, pyorrhea
• *Soft and hard palate:* Note color	Pink Torus palatinus	Lesions
• Tongue	Fissures, varicosities on under surface	Extremely dry Thrush, lesions, deviations

▓ Physical Assessment: Mouth and Tongue

Cultural Adaptations*

Steps	Normal and/or Common Findings	Significant Deviations
Inspection		
• *Lips:* Note surface integrity	African-American and Asian dimpling ≤4 mm at commissure; size and shape vary in different cultural groups	
• *Teeth:* Note size	African American larger; Asian and Native American largest; agenesis of third molars most frequent in Asians	
• *Mucosa:* Note color integrity	Hyperpigmentation	Grayish white lesion
• *Palate and lingual mandible area:*	Protuberances most common in Asians, Native Americans	May interfere with dentures
Note surface	Cleft palate and bifid uvula more common in Asians, Native Americans	May indicate cleft palate

Source: Adapted from Jarvis, 2000.

▓ Diagnostic Tests

May need to refer for:

- Dental x-rays as needed
- Biopsy of suspicious lesions
- Throat cultures
- Swallowing studies

▓ Possible Nursing Diagnoses

- Oral mucous membrane, altered
- Sensory-perceptual alteration, gustatory

- Nutrition: altered, less than body requirements
- Infection, risk for
- Aspiration, risk for

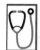

Clinical Alert

- Note severe signs of dehydration if lips, mucosa, and/or tongue are dry.
- Wear gloves to remove and clean dentures.
- Store dentures in a safe place when not in the patient's mouth.
- Excess saliva may be aspirated.
- Bright red, +4 tonsils require prompt medical attention.
- Oral lesions, gingival erythema and edema, tooth decay or abscess—refer to a dentist.
- Observe for signs of swallowing difficulties, choking during eating or drinking, coughing 15 to 30 minutes after a meal, recurrent pneumonia, and drooling.

Sample Documentation

Adult

- Oral cavity pink, moist, smooth, clean. No missing or decaying teeth. Tonsils +1, without exudate or erythema. CN IX, X, XII intact. No masses or nodules palpated.

Pediatric

- Oral cavity pink and moist. Palate intact. Hypertrophic tonsils without redness or edema. Twenty deciduous teeth present without caries.

Patient and Family Education and Home Health Notes

Adult

- Patient should brush with fluoride tooth paste at least twice a day and floss between teeth at least once a day.
- Dilantin may cause gums to bleed. Patients on this medication should cleanse with very soft brush and floss gently. They should also consider having their teeth cleaned by a dentist more frequently than every 6 months.
- Remind patients with heart disease to inform dentist of their condition.
- Remind patient to see dentist twice yearly for exam and professional cleaning. Patients who wear dentures should still see dentist every 6 months; this is necessary to check for oral cancers and problems in denture alignment. Note also that patients who have had a significant weight change should have a dentist check denture alignment.
- Remind patient to limit sweets, **including prolonged exposure to sweetened beverages.**
- Remind patient to not smoke or chew tobacco.

Pediatric

- Caution parents to avoid prolonged exposure of mouth to milk or sweetened drinks (even before eruption of teeth). If bottle is taken to bed, it should contain only water. Bottles should not be propped in crib as there is a danger of aspiration.
- Discuss food safety with parents (e.g., aspiration, danger of straws).
- Explain to parents that they should use a spoon to feed baby cereal. Cereal should not be put in a bottle (aspiration hazard).
- Before teeth emerge, parents should wipe gums gently and often with damp, soft cloth.

(Continued on following page)

- Brushing should begin with the first tooth. Parents may use infant toothbrush or a piece of gauze to clean teeth. Dental checkups should begin between ages 1 and 2; thereafter children should have checkups twice a year or yearly, as recommended by their dentist.
- Check fluoride level of drinking water for infants and children. Parents should check with dentist about taking fluoride tablets or using fluoride rinses. (Supplements are recommended if fluoride level in water <0.7 parts per million.)
- Reinforce dental hygiene guidelines for children between 7 to 10 years of age.

Geriatric

- If taste perception is decreased, encourage the use of spices such as cinnamon and garlic powder instead of extra salt and sugar.
- Explain that preventive oral care is a requirement across the life span.
- Encourage patient to brush and floss teeth daily, preferably after every meal.
- Refer patient to physician if suspect problems with swallowing.
- Denture wearers:
  - Wear dentures during waking hours to prevent atrophy of gums.
  - See dentist if dentures do not fit properly and/or cause any irritation or pain to gums.
  - Brush dentures at least daily, preferably after each meal.
  - Remove dentures at night and soak in water or a denture cleansing solution to prevent drying or warping.
  - When caring for dentures, place a washcloth in the bottom of the sink in case dentures are accidentally dropped (will help prevent possible damage to the dentures).
  - Rinse mouth thoroughly with warm water before replacing dentures in mouth after meals or in the morning.

▨ Associated Community Agencies

- Local dental or dental hygiene schools; discounted exams
- American Dental Association (free public education materials)
- American Cleft Palate–Craniofacial Association

CHAPTER **13**

Lungs and Thorax

▨ History

Adult

- Exposure to dust, chemicals and vapors, birds, asbestos, air pollutants
- Home environment, hobbies, travel
- <u>Allergies</u>: Type, response, treatments
- <u>Medications</u>: Prescription, OTC, illegal drugs
- <u>Tobacco use</u>: Type, duration, amount (packs, years), extent of passive smoking, years since quitting
- History of impaired mental status, exposure to infections
- <u>Cough</u>: Onset, type, duration, pattern, causes, severity, treatments
- *Chest pain:* Onset, duration, associated symptoms, treatments.
- *Shortness of breath (SOB):* Onset, pattern, duration, causes, treatments
- Cyanosis or pallor
- History of emphysema, cancer, tuberculosis, heart disease, asthma, chest pain, allergies, sickle cell disease, immobility, obesity

(Continued on following page)

- History of surgery trauma
- Date of last chest x-ray and tuberculosis test
- Production of blood and/or other secretions with coughing
- Sedentary lifestyle, exercise intolerance
- Family history of tuberculosis, cystic fibrosis, asthma, emphysema, malignancy

Pediatric

Infants
- Immunizations (see App., Immunization Schedule)
- Respiratory distress, cyanosis, apnea
- <u>Sudden Infant Death Syndrome (SIDS):</u> Occurrence in sibling or other family member
- Exposure to passive smoke
- History of meconium ileus
- History of prematurity or mechanical ventilation
- Possible aspiration
- Difficulty feeding

Children
- Immunizations (see App., Immunization Schedule)
- <u>Asthma history:</u> Associated factors related to episodes, treatment
- Frequent colds or congestion
- Swollen lymph nodes, sore throat, facial pain
- Night coughs

Geriatric

- History of annual influenza immunization
- History of pneumococcal vaccine
- Recent change in exertional capacity, fatigue
- Significant weight changes
- Change in number of pillows used at night
- Painful breathing: night sweats: swelling of hands, ankles; tingling of arms or legs; leg cramps at rest or with movement

(Continued on following page)

- Smoking history
- Difficulty swallowing with frequent respiratory infections
- Any shortness of breath or wheezing
- History of coughing (dry, productive, chronic)

🔲 Equipment

- Stethoscope
- Tape measure
- Pen or washable marker
- Ruler
- Drapes

🔲 Patient Preparation

- Sitting

🔲 Physical Assessment: Lungs and Thorax

Adult

Steps	Normal and/or Common Findings	Significant Deviations
Inspection		
• *Shape:* Note antero-posterior (AP) to transverse ratio	Approximately symmetrical, AP about 0.5 diameter of transverse	Barrel chest, pigeon chest, funnel chest
• Note color		Cyanosis, pallor, especially of lips, nails, gums
• *Respiration:* Note rate, rhythm, depth, pattern	12–20/min Expansion symmetrical	Distress; shallow, rapid; gasping; bradypnea, tachypnea; bulging or audible sounds; retractions

(Continued on page 174)

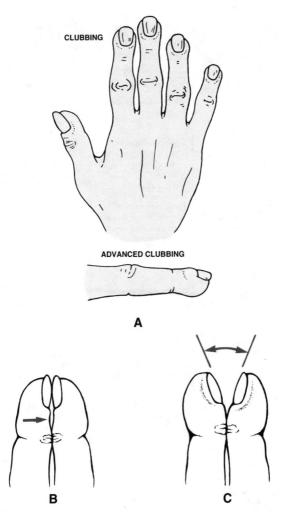

Figure 13-1 (*A*) Clubbing of fingers. (***Source:*** *Taber's Cyclopedic Medical Dictionary, 2001, ed 19, p 437, with permission.*) (*B*) Normal nails with arch illustrated by arrow. (*C*) Clubbed nails with arrow illustrating loss of arch and exaggerated angle. (***Source:*** *Adapted from Seidel et al, Mosby's Guide to Physical Examination, ed 5. Mosby, St. Louis, 2003, p 189, with permission.*)

(Continued)

Steps	Normal and/or Common Findings	Significant Deviations
Inspection (Continued)		
• *Fingers:* Note shape of nails	Uniform	Clubbing (Fig. 13–1)
• Check lips	No effort in breathing	Pursing
• Check nose	No flaring	Flaring nares
Palpation		
• *Thorax:* Note tenderness, motion, pulsation, crepitus	Approximate symmetry, firm shape, nontender, elastic motion	Pain, tenderness Crepitus (crinkly, crackles)
	No pulsations or crepitations	Friction rub (coarse vibration, usually inspiratory)
• *Tactile fremitus:* Place palmar surface of fingers on auscultation sites simultaneously; ask patient to repeat "99" while palpating; compare right and left sides	Even, symmetrical Increased over major airways, decreased over lung bases	Decreased, absent, increased asymmetrical, coarsened Crepitus
• Expansion (thumbs at 10th rib) (Fig. 13-2)	Symmetrical expansion of 2–3 in	Asymmetrical expansion <2 in
Percussion		
• *Thorax:* Compare left and right; note tone, intensity, pitch	(See Table 4-2.) Flat: Large muscles, viscera, bones *Dull:* Heart, liver *Tympany:* Stomach *Resonance:* All of lung field	Hyperresonance Dullness Hyperresonance, tympany, dullness, flatness over lung tissue
• Measure diaphragmatic excursion; percuss downward in midscapular line as patient holds deep inspiration, from resonance to dullness; mark lower border where dullness begins; ask patient to exhale completely, then percuss upward from mark to beginning of resonance; mark and measure; repeat on other side	3–5 cm; may be higher on right	No change or decrease Increased excursion

(Continued on following page)

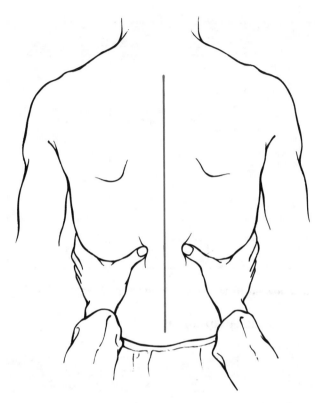

Figure 13-2 Measurement of thoracic expansion.

Steps	Normal and/or Common Findings	Significant Deviations
Auscultation • (Ask patient to breathe fairly deeply through mouth)	Vesicular, over lung field, inspiration > expiration; bronchovesicular, over	Bronchovesicular or bronchial breath sounds over peripheral lung fields

(Continued on following page)

(Continued)

Steps	Normal and/or Common Findings	Significant Deviations
Auscultation (Continued)		
• Auscultate with diaphragm, through complete inspiration and expiration, at each site, (Figs. 13-3 through 13-5) as patient crosses arms over chest and leans forward. Compare bilaterally. Note pitch, intensity, duration of inspiration and expiration (Fig. 13-6), and any adventitious sounds (Fig. 13-7)	main stem bronchi, inspiration = expiration; bronchial over trachea, inspiration < expiration	Diminished, absent, markedly increased breath sounds, adventitious sounds; crackles (rales), wheezes, gurgles (ronchi), friction
• *Cough:* Note moisture, pitch, quality, frequency	No cough	Cough with yellow, pink, brown, or gray sputum

Physical Assessment: Lungs and Thorax

Pediatric Adaptations

INFANT

Steps	Normal and/or Common Findings	Significant Deviations
Inspection		
• Note respiration rate	30–60 (newborn), 22–40 (by 1 year old)	
• *Shape:* Note chest and head circumference	Approximately equal in neonate	Unequal chest expansion
• Note AP and transverse diameter	Abdominal breathing Approximately equal	Paradoxical breathing
• Note respiratory pattern	Diaphragmatic breather	Retractions, nasal flaring, periodic breathing, apnea, grunting, stridor
Auscultation		
• Check lung fields	Loud, equal	Muffled, unequal, hyperresonant, diminished

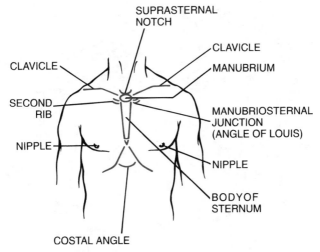

Figure 13-3 Topographic landmarks of chest.

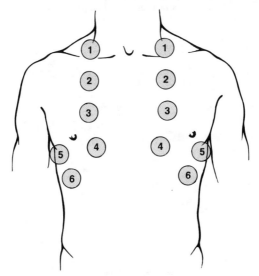

Figure 13-4 Anterior thoracic auscultation and palpation sites.

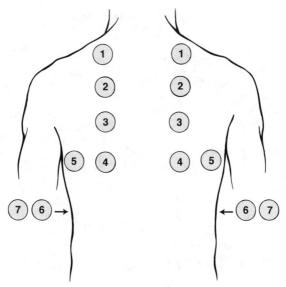

Figure 13-5 Posterior thoracic auscultation, percussion, and palpation sites.

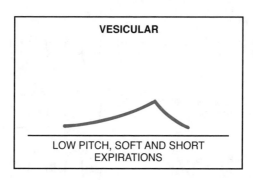

VESICULAR

LOW PITCH, SOFT AND SHORT
EXPIRATIONS

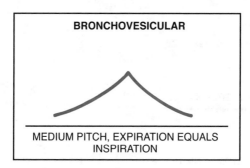

BRONCHOVESICULAR

MEDIUM PITCH, EXPIRATION EQUALS
INSPIRATION

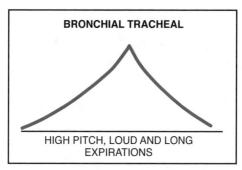

BRONCHIAL TRACHEAL

HIGH PITCH, LOUD AND LONG
EXPIRATIONS

Figure 13-6 Expected breath sounds. (*Source: Adapted from Seidel, H, et al: Mosby's Physical Examination Handbook, ed 3. Mosby, St. Louis, 2003, p. 98, with permission.*)

CRACKLES:

FINE CRACKLES
(RALES)

MEDIUM CRACKLES
(RALES)

COARSE CRACKLES
(RALES)

WHEEZES

SIBILANT WHEEZE

SONOROUS WHEEZE
(RHONCHI)

PLEURAL FRICTION RUB

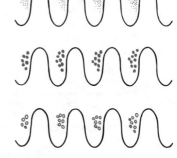
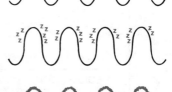
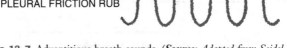

Figure 13-7 Adventitious breath sounds. (***Source:*** *Adapted from Seidel, H, et al: Mosby's Physical Examination Handbook, ed 3. Mosby, St. Louis, 2003, p. 99, with permission.*)

🔹 Physical Assessment: Lungs and Thorax

Pediatric Adaptations

CHILD

Steps	Normal and/or Common Findings	Significant Deviations
Inspection • Shape	Should approximate adult shape, uniform	Barrel chest Pectus carinatum Pectus excavatum
• Rate	Approximately: 26 by age 4 20 by age 10 16 by age 16	

🔹 Physical Assessment: Lungs and Thorax

Geriatric Adaptations

Steps	Normal and/or Common Findings	Significant Deviations
Inspection • *Thoracic spine:* Note curvature, angles	Essentially straight	Marked dorsal curvature, kyphosis, increased AP diameter of chest
• Assess chest expansion		Diminished

🔲 Physical Assessment: Lungs and Thorax

Cultural Adaptations

Steps	Normal and/or Common Findings	Significant Deviations
Inspection • Note position while breathing		Arching back to ease dyspnea in sickle cell crisis
Auscultation • Look for signs of cor pulmonale		Productive cough, exertional dyspnea, wheezing, fatigue, dependent edema, weak rapid pulse

🔲 Diagnostic Tests

May need to refer for:

• Chest x-ray
• TB test
• Culture and sensitivity of sputum
• Modified barium swallow

🔲 Possible Nursing Diagnoses

• Airway clearance, ineffective
• Breathing pattern, ineffective
• Suffocation, risk for
• Tissue perfusion, altered: cardiopulmonary
• Gas exchange, impaired
• Infection, risk for

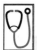 Clinical Alert

- Persistent or paroxysmal cough
- Cyanosis
- Air hunger, dyspnea
- Hemoptysis
- Stridor

Sample Documentation

Color pink without cyanosis or pallor. Respiration 16, regular, even depth. Chest equal symmetrically; AP diameter is half transverse. Tactile fremitus and thoracic expansion symmetrical and equal. All lung fields resonant equally. Vesicular sounds throughout; no adventitious sounds auscultated.

Patient and Family Education and Home Health Notes

General

- Educate all patients about need for annual influenza vaccination.

Adult

- Educate about smoking hazards, indoor pollution, exposure to respiratory irritants.
- Offer literature on quitting smoking, effective breathing patterns and coughing awareness, controlled breathing techniques.
- Be sure college students have had second measles-mumps-rubella vaccination.

(Continued on following page)

Pediatric

- Educate parents regarding importance of immunizations.
- Instruct parents in risks associated with passive smoking.
- Discuss smoking with adolescents. Educate about smoking hazards.
- Refer for smoking cessation, as appropriate.
- Instruct parents in use of vaporizer or humidifier.
- Educate parents on importance of handwashing to prevent spread of viral and bacterial infections.
- Caution parents about the risks of infants and small children aspirating foreign objects, foods, and toy parts.
- Explain hazards of choking associated with adding cereal to bottles and/or propping bottles in the crib.
- Encourage parents to take cardiopulmonary resuscitation (CPR) class.
- Discuss swimming safety issues.
- Instruct parents to position infant on back or side unless prohibited by other medical problems.

Geriatric

- Instruct patients to avoid environments where there are persons with respiratory infections.
- Instruct patients to avoid noxious fumes.
- Note that infection may occur without a major increase in temperature or presence of a severe cough.
- Note that most older persons should have pneumococcal and influenza vaccinations. Initial vaccination at age 65 and recommended revaccination every 5–6 years and thereafter. Influenza vaccinations are neces-

(Continued on following page)

sary yearly. If patient is immunosuppressed or has a chronic disease, he or she may need influenza or pneumococcal vaccinations before age 65. Health-care workers should receive influenza vaccinations before age 65.

- Raising the head and shoulders on several pillows can help persons breathe better when they feel dyspneic.
- Refer patients to physician in case of persistent cough.

Clinical Alert

Refer any person with a persistent or productive cough, new or increased dyspnea, orthopnea, or painful breathing.

Associated Community Agencies

- American Lung Association: Health promotion information, better breathing club, asthma camp
- Office on Smoking and Health: Information and publications
- American Cancer Society: Provides hospital beds and other adaptive aids for cancer patients, helps finance prescriptions for cancer treatment, health promotion information
- Cystic Fibrosis Foundation
- National Foundation for Asthma

CHAPTER

Breasts and Axillae

History

- Age at menarche, menopause
- Age during pregnancies, breast-feeding
- Use of hormonal medications, oral contraceptives, hormone replacement therapy
- <u>Breast self-examination:</u> How often, method used
- <u>Mammogram:</u> Date, findings
- Breast surgery, trauma, or disease
- <u>Change in breast:</u> Lumps, discharge, shape, skin, lesions, erythema, swelling, tenderness, change in position of nipple, nipple discharge or inversion, relationship of breast changes to menses
- <u>Breast cancer, self, family:</u> Age at diagnosis, treatment, response
- <u>Lumps:</u> Size, location, how long, tenderness, relationship to menses
- Rash or eczema on nipples
- Fat and caffeine intake
- Risk factors for breast cancer:
  - Over age 40, female
  - Early menarche, late menopause, chronically irregular menses untreated
  - Nulliparity
  - Over age 30 with first pregnancy
  - Previous breast cancer
  - Ovarian, uterine, or bowel cancer
  - Medications to suppress lactation
  - Breast cancer in mother, sister, aunt, grandmother, daughter
  - High intake of dietary fat
  - Postmenopausal weight gain *(Continued on following page)*

- Age at thelarche
- *Adolescent boys:* Unilateral or bilateral enlargement of breasts

Geriatric

- Prescription medications that may cause gynecomastia in older men
- Breast self-examinations
- Recent changes in breast characteristics
- Injury to breast tissue

Equipment

- Small pillow
- Measuring tape
- Small sheet or towel

Patient Preparation

Adult

- Patient should be sitting and may need to stand and bend forward.
- Maintain privacy.

Pediatric

- Explain normal process of physical and sexual development.
- Tell child findings are normal.

▉ Physical Assessment: Breasts and Axillae

Adult

Steps	Normal and/or Common Findings	Significant Deviations
Inspection		
• Repeat in three positions for women, sitting position only for men; sitting, arms at side; sitting, arms raised over head; sitting, hand on hips, pushing in; if breasts are very large, have patient stand, bend forward at waist; inspect for shape and contour		
• Shape	Conical to pendulous	Marked difference in contour
• Size, symmetry	Generally equal	Marked differences
• Contour	Symmetrical	Retraction, dimpling, flattening
• Color	Light, striae Darkened areola	Redness
• Venous pattern	Symmetrical, faint	Superficial dilation, asymmetrically increased pattern
• Texture	Smooth, soft	Lesions, peau d'orange appearance
• Nipple, areolar tissue	Lifetime inversion, Montgomery tubercles, supernumerary nipples	Retraction, deviation, rashes, discharge, recent inversion
Palpation		
• *Repeat in two positions for women:* Sitting arms at sides; supine, small pillow under shoulder of side being palpated; omit supine position for men; follow either clock or wedge pattern, using pads of three fingers (Figs. 14–1 through 14–3); palpate breast and axillae		

(Continued on following page)

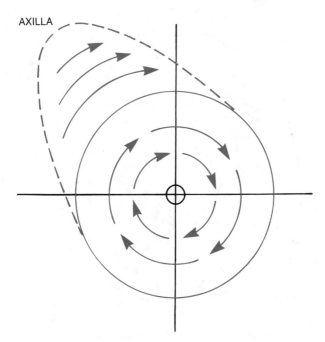

AXILLA

Figure 14–1 A palpation method for the breast and tail of Spence.

Steps	Normal and/or Common Findings	Significant Deviations
• Consistency • Tenderness	Varies Tender if premenstrual	Thickening, masses Pain
• *Nodules:* Note location, size, shape, consistency, delimitation, mobility, tenderness	None	Masses, areas of induration
• *Nipples:* Gently compress	No discharge	Discharge

(Continued on following page)

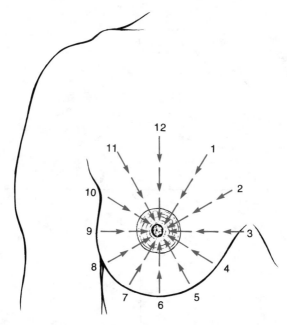

Figure 14–2 Clock pattern of breast examination.

(Continued)

Steps	Normal and/or Common Findings	Significant Deviations
Palpation (Continued) • *Lymph nodes:* Lateral, subscapular, pectoral, central; note presence, location, size, delimitation, shape, consistency, mobility, tenderness	None	Palpable

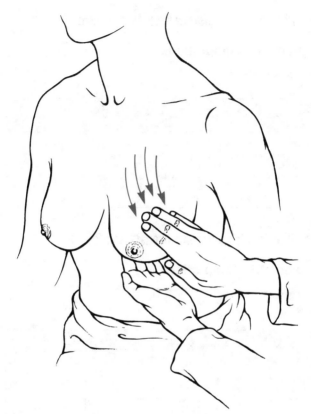

Figure 14–3 Bimanual palpation of the breast: Technique used for large, pendulous breasts.

■ Physical Assessment: Breasts and Axillae

Pediatric Adaptations

INFANT

Steps	Normal and/or Common Findings	Significant Deviations
Inspection • *Breasts:* Note size, discharge	Nonpalpable, no discharge. Engorgement <1.5 cm, scant milky discharge in newborns; supernumerary nipples	

■ Physical Assessment: Breasts and Axillae

Pediatric Adaptations

CHILD

Steps	Normal and/or Common Findings	Significant Deviations
Inspection • *Breasts:* Note size, symmetry	Breast development after age 8; may be asymmetrical (Table 14–1)	
Palpation • *Breast:* Note tenderness, masses	Boys may have small, tender breast buds Tender	Masses Gynecomastia

Table 14-1

Stages of Secondary Sexual Characteristics: Female Breast Development

Stage	Female Breast Development
I	*Preadolescent:* Elevation of papilla only
II	*Small breast bud:* Elevation of breast and papilla as small mound with enlarging areola
III	Areola and breast tissue enlarged
IV	*Areola and papilla form secondary:* Contour develops simultaneous mound on breast; nipple and areola above level of rest of breast
V	Maturity: Nipple only projects, areola receding to general breast level

Source: Data from Tanner, JM: Fetus into Man: Physical Growth From Conception to Maturity. Harvard University Press, Cambridge, MA, 1990.

 Physical Assessment: Breasts and Axillae

Geriatric Adaptations

Steps	Normal and/or Common Findings	Significant Deviations
Inspection		
• *Breasts:* Note size, shape, lesions, color, nodules	Loose, atrophied, pendulous	Redness, irritation under breast, dimpling, masses
• *Nipples:* Note size, direction	Flat, small	Dimpling, recent or new inversion, masses, discharge

Diagnostic Tests

May need to refer for:
* Mammogram
* Biopsy

Possible Nursing Diagnoses

* Tissue integrity, impaired
* Body image disturbance
* Self-esteem disturbance
* Anxiety

Clinical Alert

Refer any suspicious lump, skin changes, dimpling, new nipple inversion or nipple discharge, or unusual breast discomfort.

Sample Documentation

Adult

* Breast symmetrical, small, without lesions: texture smooth. No discharge or tenderness of nipple or areola. Nipples everted bilaterally. No masses or tenderness palpable in any region of breast or tail of Spence. No axillary or epitrochlear nodes palpable.

Infant

* Nipples symmetrical. No discharge. No masses.

Child

* Tanner stage II. No discharge. No masses or tenderness.

🔖 Patient and Family Education and Home Health Notes

Adult

- Assess patient's understanding of breast cancer, history, prevention, and early detection.
- Instruct both male and female patients on breast self-examination (BSE) (Fig. 14-4)
- Explain importance of regular breast exam performed by a health professional.
- Explain how a high-fat diet is related to an increased risk for breast cancer.
- Explain relationship of large intake of caffeine and fat and breast cancer.
- Explain importance of mammogram and suggested schedule: once between ages 35 and 40, every year or every other year between ages 40 and 50, and every year after age 50 (more frequently if at risk).
- Explain incidence of recovery related to cancer.
- Encourage questions.

Pediatric

Infants
- Explain influence of maternal hormones to parents if infant has palpable breast tissue.

Children
- Explain patterns of breast development.
- Reassure adolescent boys with breast enlargement that condition is temporary.
- Teach BSE.

Geriatric

- Explain the importance of monthly BSE at set date every month after menopause (e.g., the first day of the month).
- Encourage patient to continue mammogram screening.

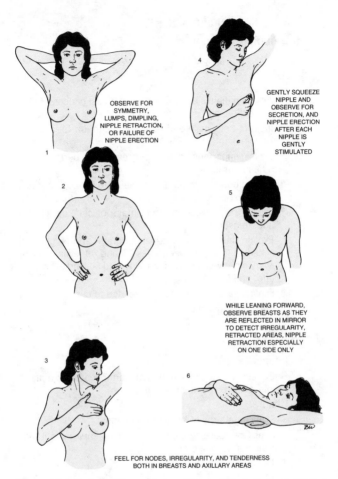

Figure 14-4 Breast self-examination. (*Source*: *Taber's Cyclopedic Medical Dictionary, 2001, ed 19, p 289, with permission.*)

▪ Associated Community Agencies

- American Cancer Society

CHAPTER **15**

Cardiovascular System

 History

Adult

- <u>Tobacco use:</u> Age started, type, amount (pack-years), duration, years since quitting
- <u>Exercise habits:</u> Amount, type, duration, response
- <u>Nutrition:</u> Usual diet: fat, salt, cholesterol, calorie intake
- <u>Weight:</u> Recent change, overweight and obesity. See Chapter 5 for guidelines and appendixes
- <u>Alcohol use:</u> Amount, frequency
- Stress management skills, ability, and methods used to relax; response to pressure, anger
- Self or family history of heart disease, diabetes, rheumatic fever, hyperlipidemia, hypertension, early deaths, congenital heart defects
- <u>Presence or history of chest pain:</u> Onset, duration, severity, characteristics, associated symptoms, treatment, response
- Shortness of breath (SOB)
- Recent increase in fatigue, inability to complete usual activities
- Dyspnea, orthopnea
- Cough
- <u>Leg cramps:</u> Onset (daily activities, awake at night), duration, characteristics
- <u>Extremities:</u> Coldness, tingling, numbness, cyanosis, lesions, varicosities, slowed healing, edema
- <u>Medication use:</u> Prescription and OTC
- Syncope

(Continued on following page)

Pediatric

Infants
- Unusual fatigue, effort, or diaphoresis especially when feeding
- Circumoral cyanosis
- Coordination problems
- Generalized cyanosis (especially when crying)
- Breathing changes
- Mother's health during pregnancy (rubella: first trimester, unexplained fever, drug use)

Children
- For people 2 to 20 years old, use a body mass index (BMI) for age chart for the appropriate gender and plot the BMI versus the child's age.
- <u>Unusual fatigue:</u> Amount, degree, activity level, need for rest, naps longer than expected
- Assumption of squatting or knee-chest position when playing
- Difficulty feeding
- Complaints of leg pain, joint pain, headache
- Nosebleeds
- Frequent streptococcal infections or sore throat with fever
- Headaches

Geriatric

- Chest pain, chest pressure, chest tightness
- Unusual fatigue, increased need for rest
- <u>Orthopnea:</u> Excessive number of pillows
- SOB, dyspnea, coughing, wheezing
- Dizziness, syncope, palpitations, confusion
- Use of cardiac or hypertensive medications
- Pounding heart with stress
- <u>Dietary history:</u> Intake of potassium, cholesterol, caffeine
- Nocturia

(Continued on following page)

- <u>Foot and leg edema:</u> Tightness of shoes at end of day; check for pitting or non-pitting edema, for calf tenderness to rule out deep vein thrombosis (DVT) and check if skin is shiny and taut
- Change in exercise level
- Use of restrictive clothing
- SOB at night
- Peripheral vascular complaints such as coldness, decreased pain sensation, exaggerated response to cold, lower extremity fatigue/discomfort that worsens with walking or resting leg pain

Cultural

- Sickle cell disease; associated subjective signs of pain, lethargy, dyspnea, low-grade fever

🔹 Equipment

- Stethoscope with diaphragm and bell
- Centimeter ruler
- Light
- Scale

The assessment of blood pressure (BP) is a part of assessing the cardiac system, but it is found in the vital signs section.

🔹 Patient Preparation

Adult

- Remove clothing: drape well for warmth and privacy.
- Positions: Primarily sitting: also supine, left lateral recumbent, standing.

(Continued on following page)

- A quiet child and a quiet environment are important.
- Use a pacifier to quiet an infant.
- Allow parent to hold child.

■ Physical Assessment: Heart

Adult

Steps	Normal and/or Common Findings	Significant Deviations
Inspection • Precordium movement with tangential lighting • Jugular vein • General muscle mass	Slight apical impulse at midclavicular line (MCL), 5th intercostal space (ICS)	Marked pulsations; often not visible; impulse visible in more than one ICS or lateral to MCL; pulsations in other locations; heaves, lifts
Palpation • Lightly palpate precordium; note location, strength of apical impulse • Palpate carotid and apical impulse simultaneously	Mild sensation palpable at 5th left intercostal space (LICS), MCL Synchronous pulses	Thrills, pulsations Palpable in radius >1–2 cm or significantly to left or right of MCL or upward
Auscultation • Auscultate in each of five areas (Fig. 15–1); sitting, with diaphragm; supine, with both diaphragm and bell • Note rate, rhythm, location, and nature of S_1, S_2	Synchronous pulses Normal sinus rhythm; S_1 loudest at apex; S_2 at base; splitting of S_1 usually heard at left lower sternal border (tricuspid area); splitting of S_2 usually heard during inspiration at 2nd or 3rd left intercostal space (LICS)	S_3, S_4 audible at apex on inspiration Extra heart sounds such as clicks, snaps, friction rubs

(Continued on following page)

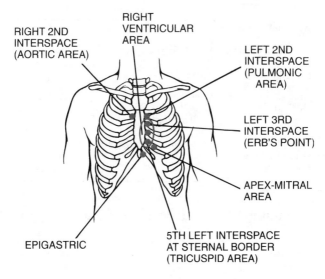

Figure 15-1 Cardiac auscultation and palpation sites.

Steps	Normal and/or Common Findings	Significant Deviations
• Auscultate along left sternal border at 2nd and 3rd ICS (pulmonic area) with diaphragm as patient leans forward; with patient in left lateral recumbent position, auscultate at 5th LICS (mitral area) with bell	No murmurs	Murmurs; note if increased on inspiration or expiration, with Valsalva maneuver, with elevation of legs, or if associated with diastole or systole (Table 15–1)

Table 15-1

Classification of Murmurs

Classification	Murmur
Grade I	Faint
Grade II	Heard fairly well in all positions
Grade III	Loud, no thrills
Grade IV	Loud, with a thrill
Grade V	Very loud, easily palpable thrill
Grade VI	May be heard without a stethoscope; thrill present

◼ Physical Assessment: Peripheral Circulation

Adult

Steps	Normal and/or Common Findings	Significant Deviations
Inspection		
• Skin of extremities: Note color, continuity, edema, vascularity	Pink, no edema, no lesions	Cyanosis, lesions, ulcers, varicosities, edema, rubor
Palpation		
• Palpate carotid pulses (one at a time)	Symmetrical, rate 60–100 beats per minute, regular rhythm	Unequal, marked bradycardia, tachycardia, arrhythmias such as bigeminal pulse, alternating pulse, bounding or absent pulse
• Palpate peripheral pulses bilaterally (Fig. 15–2):		
• Brachial		
• Radial		
• Femoral		
• Popliteal		
• Dorsalis pedis		
• Posterior tibial Note rate, rhythm, strength, symmetry; compare side to side		

(Continued on following page)

Steps	Normal and/or Common Findings	Significant Deviations
• Palpate extremities; note temperature, tenderness, turgor, texture, hair growth, nails, varicosities, lesions, capillary refill time	Warm; nontender; firm without edema; equal, fine hair growth; no lesions or varicosities, capillary refill <2 seconds	Cool, tender, pitting edema (0 to +4), absence of hair, varicose veins
• Measure jugular venous pressure; place patient in supine position with 45-degree elevation of head and shoulders; observe jugular pulsation; with centimeter ruler, measure between highest point of jugular pulsation and angle of Louis (Fig. 15–3); mark the jugular pressure point with a straightedge for ease of measuring; repeat on other side	≤2 cm; usually absent on persons <age 50	>2 cm
Auscultation		
• *Auscultate with bell:* Temporal, carotid	No audible sounds	Bruits

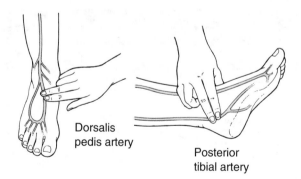

A. Palpation of dorsalis   B. Palpation of posterior
   pedis artery   tibial pulse

Figure 15-2 Palpation of peripheral pulses.

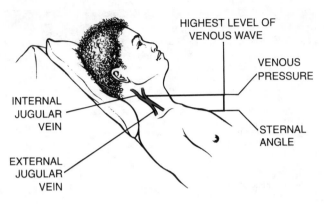

Figure 15-3 Inspection of jugular vein.

Physical Assessment: Heart and Peripheral Circulation

Pediatric Adaptations

INFANT

Steps	Normal and/or Common Findings	Significant Deviations
Inspection • *Apical impulse:* Note location	4th LICS medial to MCL (<5 years old)	On right side may indicate situs inversus, heave
Palpation • Apical impulse • *Femoral and brachial pulses:* Note symmetry	Equal bilaterally	Thrills Bounding Absent or weak in lower extremities
• Note capillary refill	1–2 seconds	>2 seconds
Auscultation • *Heart sounds:* Note rate, rhythm, location, nature of S_1, S_2, S_3	Sinus arrhythmia	Machinelike continuous murmur, bradycardia, tachycardia

◼ Physical Assessment: Heart and Peripheral Circulation

Pediatric Adaptations

CHILD

Steps	Normal and/or Common Findings	Significant Deviations

Inspection
• Apical impulse medial to left MCL at 4th ICS in child <5 years old
	Heart rate:
	  1 year old: 80–140
	  3 years old: 80–120
	  5 years old: 75–110
	  10 years old: 70–100
	Sinus arrhythmia	

Auscultation • *Heart sounds:* Sitting and supine	Splitting of S$_2$ at apex; innocent murmurs, grade 3 or less, present in systole; varying with respirations, found along left sternal border with child supine	No splitting of S$_2$ during inspiration
• BP: all four extremities	Equal	Discrepancy between BP in upper and lower extremities may be indicative of coarctation of the aorta

◼ Physical Assessment: Heart and Peripheral Circulation

Geriatric Adaptations

Steps	Normal and/or Common Findings	Significant Deviations
Inspection • Feet, toes, extremities	Varicose veins may appear when legs are in dependent position; veins should collapse when elevated; nails thicken; hair thins	Rubor, lesions, marked edema, persistent cyanosis, venous stasis, brown skin, color changes, marked pallor, delayed color return, *resting* leg pain, nonhealing ulcers, pain (positive Homans' sign), redness, tenderness along superficial vein
Auscultation • BP	Pulse pressure may reach 100	Varies, serial readings >120/80 (prehypertension) >140/90 (hypertension)
• Heart sounds	Murmurs may be benign, attributable to stiffened valves; S$_4$ may be attributable to decreased left ventricle compliance	Loud murmurs, pericardial friction rub, arrhythmia, or gallop
Palpation • Extremities	Pulses may be difficult to locate	Absent or asymmetrical peripheral pulses
• Heart		Displaced PMI, thrill

Physical Assessment: Heart and Peripheral Circulation

Cultural Adaptations

Steps	Normal and/or Common Findings	Significant Deviations
Inspection • *Extremities:* Note dependent edema, capillary refill • Hair growth on feet, hands	Smooth, hairless	Swelling, pale nail beds may indicate impending sickle cell crisis
Auscultation • *Heart sounds:* Note rate, estimated heart size, murmurs		Tachycardia, cardiomegaly; systolic and/or diastolic murmurs, which may be indicative of impending sickle cell crisis
• BP		Hypertension: Assess significance

Diagnostic Tests

May need to refer for:
• Cardiac catheterization
• Exercise stress test
• Chest x-ray
• Enzyme studies
• Electrocardiogram (ECG)
• Complete blood count (CBC)
• Triglycerides
• Cholesterol
• Echocardiogram

🔖 Possible Nursing Diagnoses

- Nutrition: altered, risk for more than body requirements
- Skin integrity, impaired, risk for,
- Cardiac output, decreased
- Tissue perfusion, altered: peripheral
- Activity intolerance (specify level), risk for
- Fatigue
- Sensory perceptual alterations (specify)
- Self-care deficit (specify)
- Role performance, altered [learning need] (specify)
- Knowledge deficit [learning need] (specify)

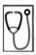

Clinical Alert

- Report any unusual heart sounds.
- Report decreased circulation, venous insufficiency, or lower extremity ulcers.
- Report chest pain, dyspnea, or marked hypertension.

🔖 Sample Documentation

BP 126/72, apical pulse 80, heart RRR, without murmurs, gallop, or rub. PMI at 5th ICS, MCL. Extremities symmetrically warm, pink, without edema or clubbing; peripheral pulses equally palpable +2 (carotid, radial, femoral, popliteal, posterior tibial, dorsalis pedis).

Patient and Family Education and Home Health Notes

Adult

- Discuss risk factors of heart disease.
- Explain principles of aerobic exercise and a low-fat, low-cholesterol, and low-sodium diet in prevention of heart disease and hypertension.
- Offer guidelines on stress management, including minimal use of caffeine, tobacco, and alcohol.
- Explain importance of unrestricted circulation and regular exercise. Instruct patient to avoid sitting for prolonged periods, to elevate legs if necessary to sit for prolonged periods, to avoid tight clothing, especially socks and hosiery, and to avoid crossing the legs while sitting.
- Explain importance of having BP checked every 2 years or more often if elevated.
- Explain importance of having cholesterol checked every 5 years or more often if elevated.

Pediatric

- Explain to parents the importance of lifetime habits for good nutrition and exercise.
- Teach that school children need an hour of vigorous daily activity.
- Stress the need to include fats in the infant's and toddler's diet and the need to reduce fats in the child's diet.
- Discuss possible need for additional iron during infancy and adolescence.

Geriatric

- Instruct patient to check with primary care provider (PCP) before starting an exercise program. Stop exercising when fatigued.
- Review medications and provide appropriate education. Explain the need to take medication as prescribed and discuss possible side effects.
- Teach the importance of proper foot and skin care.

(Continued on following page)

Geriatric   *(Continued)*

- Report any new SOB, edema, and/or weight gain to physician.
- Monitor blood pressure and pulse rate as instructed by PCP.
- Teach patient how to check BP and pulse rate.
- Instruct the patient to follow the regimen prescribed by his or her physician for any chronic diseases and to keep follow-up appointments.
- Provide information about programs to help people stop smoking.
- Instruct patient to reduce saturated fat and sodium intake.
- Suggest that patient use stress reduction techniques such as deep breathing, progressive muscle relaxation, and guided imagery and reduce stressful stimuli from lifestyle.

Associated Community Agencies

- American Heart Association: Health promotion literature, CPR classes.
- American Red Cross: CPR classes
- National Heart, Lung, and Blood Institute: Information

CHAPTER **16**

Abdomen

History

Adult

- Appetite
- Diet recall for the past 24 hours
- Dysphagia

(Continued on following page)

- Weight gain or loss
- Use of alcohol, tobacco, caffeine: Duration, amount, frequency
- Bowel and/or bladder routines, problems
- <u>Indigestion, nausea, vomiting, diarrhea, pain, jaundice, flatulence, incontinence:</u> Causes, frequency, treatments
- <u>Pain:</u> Type, predisposing factors, time, relationship to eating
- Medications for bowel, indigestion
- History of hepatitis, ulcer, arthritis
- History of gastrointestinal diagnostic tests, surgery
- History of eating disorders
- Hepatitis vaccination

Pediatric

- Congenital anomalies
- Jaundice
- Pain or paroxysmal fussiness and intense crying
- Frequent spitting up
- Projectile vomiting
- Constipation, encopresis, crying while urinating, frequency of urinary tract infections (UTIs)
- Introduction to new foods
- Type and methods of feeding
- Parental concerns
- Milk intake
- Pica intake
- History of eating disorders
- Diarrhea, colic, failure to gain weight, weight loss

Geriatric

- Abdominal pain, specifying whether the pain is associated with eating
- Excessive belching, bloating, flatulence
- Changes in appetite (especially a decrease in appetite)
- Nausea, vomiting, diarrhea

(Continued on following page)

Geriatric   *(Continued)*

- Hemorrhoids, changes in bowel habits
- Rectal bleeding, pain, or itching; hernia
- Bowel habits (constipation, incontinence, or loose stools, use of laxatives)
- Change in appearance of stools (tarry, bloody, pencil-shaped)
- Nutritional assessment: Appetite and/or intake, any functional problems interfering with shopping for food or meal preparation, available external support for meal preparation, weight loss, albumin and total protein levels, financial barriers to good nutrition, swallowing difficulties, difficulty chewing, or mouth discomfort

Cultural

- <u>History of familial Mediterranean fever:</u> periodic peritonitis
- Travel experiences, especially exposure to parasites

Equipment

- Ink pen
- Stethoscope
- Tape measure
- Gloves

Patient Preparation

- Have patient empty bladder.
- Have patient lie on back with knees bent.
- Have parent hold child <3 years old on lap if child is unable to lie on back.
- Place child's hand under yours during palpation if child is ticklish.

🔲 Physical Assessment: Abdomen

Adult

Steps	Normal and/or Common Findings	Significant Deviations
Inspection		
• *Shape:* Note symmetry, contour	Flat, rounded	Protuberant scaphoid (Fig. 16–1), asymmetry, masses
• Check color	Same as or lighter than other areas	Redness, cyanosis, jaundice, lesions (see Integumentary System)
• *Surface:* Note motion (respiratory, digestive)		Circulatory pulsations
		Dilated veins
Auscultation		
• Lightly place warmed stethoscope (diaphragm) over diaphragm		
• *Abdomen:* Note bowel sounds; pitch, volume, frequency in four quadrants (Fig. 16–2)	Bowel sounds, 5–35/min	Absent bowel sounds (after 5 minutes' continuous listening), absence of borborygmus
	No vascular sounds	Bruits, hums, rubs
• Assess aortic, renal, femoral, arteries		
Percussion		
• *Four quadrants:* Note percussion sounds (see Table 4–2)	Tympany, dullness	
• *Liver:* Note size; on right midcostal line (MCL), percuss upward from below umbilicus to dullness (lower border); mark with pen at dullness; move up to lung resonance and percuss downward in MCL to dullness (upper border of liver); mark at dullness and measure (Fig. 16–3)	6–12 cm	Enlarged >12 cm or <6 cm

(Continued on page 215)

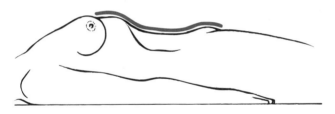

Figure 16-1 Scaphoid abdomen.

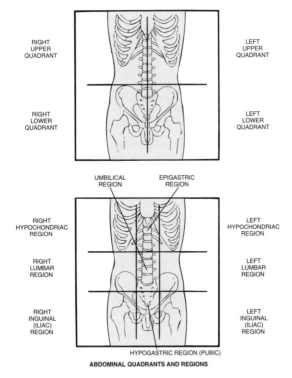

ABDOMINAL QUADRANTS AND REGIONS

Figure 16-2 Abdominal quadrants and regions. (***Source:*** *Adapted from Taber's Cyclopedic Medical Dictionary, 2001, ed 19; p 4, with permission.*)

(Continued)

Steps	Normal and/or Common Findings	Significant Deviations
Percussion (Continued)		
• *Liver scratch test:* Place stethoscope over liver; scratch skin surface lightly from middle of liver out toward periphery; sound will diminish significantly when passing liver borders		
• *Spleen:* Note size; percuss on left side, distal to MCL (have patient turn slightly to right side)	Should be between ribs 6 and 10	Enlarged
• *Abdominal wall:* Palpate deeply (Fig. 16–4); check four quadrants (see Fig. 16–2)		Tenderness, masses, bulges
• *Note organs:* Liver, spleen, kidneys		
• *Aorta*	Palpable in midline	Prominent lateral pulsation
• Measure the waist circumference: With the patient standing, palpate the uppermost border of the right iliac crest; just above this landmark, make a horizontal mark and then cross it with a vertical mark along the midaxillary line; use this mark to position the measuring tape around the patient, making sure that the tape is parallel to the floor; the tape should be snug, but not compressing the skin; take the measurement during normal respiration	Men: ≤ 102 cm (40 in) Women: ≤ or = 88 cm (35 in)	Men: > 102 cm (40 in) Women: > 88 cm (35 in)

(Continued on following page)

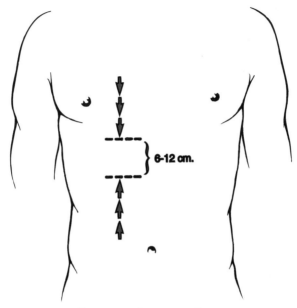

Figure 16-3 Percussion of liver.

(Continued)

Steps	Normal and/or Common Findings	Significant Deviations
Palpation Use the palmar surface of extended fingers • *Abdominal wall:* Palpate lightly	No tenderness, pain, masses	Tenderness, rigidity, nodules

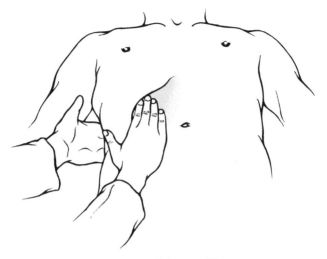

Figure 16-4 Palpation of liver.

Physical Assessment: Abdomen

Pediatric Adaptations

NEONATE

Steps	Normal and/or Common Findings	Significant Deviations
Inspection • Shape of abdomen	Flat immediately following birth, then prominent and protuberant	Scaphoid abdomen in neonate may indicate diaphragmatic hernia Loose, wrinkled skin
• Umbilical cord	Presence of two umbilical arteries, thick white or cream-colored walls, and one vein	One umbilical artery Gastroschisis

▣ Physical Assessment: Abdomen

Pediatric Adaptations

INFANT

Steps	Normal and/or Common Findings	Significant Deviations
Inspection		
• Shape of abdomen	Protuberant because of the underdeveloped musculature	Umbilical or ventral herniations: diastasis recti; weakness of the musculature
• Motion		Visible reverse peristalsis
• *Umbilical stump:* Note color, odor	Stump falls off 10–15 days after birth	Signs of infection; foul odor
Auscultation		
• Bowel sounds	Listen every 10–30 seconds	Absent (after 5 minutes' continuous listening), hyperactive
Palpation		
• Have infant supine; place folded blanket under infant's knees and hips to elevate feet and relax abdominal muscles; because infants have limited verbal ability, observe infant for facial cues indicating discomfort		
• Liver	1-2 cm below right costal margin (RCM)	Enlarged
• Spleen tip		Tenderness, mass, difficult to assess
• Bladder		
• Descending colon		
Percussion		
• Bladder	May reach level of umbilicus at times; children have more tympany than adults because of presence of more air in intestines	

🔲 Physical Assessment: Abdomen

Pediatric Adaptations

CHILD

Steps	Normal and/or Common Findings	Significant Deviations
Inspection • Assess shape of abdomen	Abdomen should be protuberant when child is standing, flat when lying supine	Distention Distended veins
• *Abdomen:* Note pulsations		Marked aortic pulsation
Palpation • Place child's hand under yours to prevent tickling		Child keeps knees drawn up, abdominal pain, splinting abdomen
• Assess liver edge	Should be < 3 cm below costal margin	Enlarged liver
• Check bladder	May be palpated just above the symphysis pubis in the pre-schooler	
• Check spleen tip	1-2 cm: Below LCM	Enlarged spleen
• Assess lower poles of both kidneys	Rarely palpable	

🔲 Physical Assessment: Abdomen

Geriatric Adaptations

Steps	Normal and/or Common Findings	Significant Deviations
Inspection • Contour	Sagging, rounded because of loss of muscle tone and an increase in fat deposits	Marked distention or concavity

(Continued on following page)

(Continued)

Steps	Normal and/or Common Findings	Significant Deviations
Auscultation • Assess bowel sounds	Diminished peristalsis Hyperactive with large doses of laxatives	Absent after listening for 5 minutes
Palpation • (Deeper and firmer palpation may be required to elicit pain or rebound tenderness) • *Liver:* Note size	May be decreased, but may extend 2–3 cm below right costal margin because of enlarged lung fields	Markedly enlarged
• Check aorta	May be dilated	Bruits

🔲 Physical Assessment: Abdomen

Cultural Adaptations

Steps	Normal and/or Common Findings	Significant Deviations
Palpation • Note organ size		Hepatomegaly, hyposplenism, or splenomegaly (sickle cell disease indications)

🔲 Diagnostic Tests

May need to refer for:
• CBC
• Bilirubin

- Electrolytes
- Barium enema
- Stool guaiac
- Hepatic panel (liver enzymes)
- Endogastroduodenoscopy, colonoscopy, flexible sigmoi-doscopy
- Abdominal ultrasound or CT scan

Possible Nursing Diagnoses

- Constipation, perceived or risk of
- Diarrhea
- Urinary elimination, altered patterns of
- Fluid volume deficit, risk for
- Nutrition: altered, less than or more than body requirements
- Sleep pattern disturbance

Clinical Alert

- Absence of bowel sounds
- Palpable masses
- Enlarged spleen, liver
- Acute abdominal pain, nausea, or vomiting
- Changes in bowel habits or blood in stool
- Difficulty swallowing
- Dyspepsia

Sample Documentation

Adult

- Abdomen smooth, rounded, nontender. Bowel sounds active in all quadrants. Liver size approximately 10 cm at MCL, not palpable. No organomegaly or masses palpated. No visible aortic pulsation and no bruits auscultated.

(Continued on following page)

- Pot-bellied appearance of abdomen. Soft. Bowel sounds present in all four quadrants. No hepatomegaly, splenomegaly, masses, or tenderness.

Patient and Family Education and Home Health Notes

- Explain the dynamics of a balanced diet in terms of calories, height, and activity. One formula, for example, that expresses the interrelationships among these factors is as follows: Ideal weight × 13-15-20 activity factor. Another useful formula to give to patients is the following: ≤30 percent fats (10 percent each: saturated, monounsaturated, polyunsaturated); cholesterol <300 mg daily; 12 percent protein; 48 percent carbohydrates; ≤10 percent refined sugar; and ≤5 g of salt daily.
- Review with the patient the Food Guide Pyramid (App. N).
- Review weight status, body mass index (BMI), what it means, and health consequences of overweight and obesity.
- Review waist circumference and explain that this measure is used to assess abdominal fat. Explain that excess abdominal fat increases the risk for obesity-related diseases, especially Type 2 diabetes.
- Teach that losing a small amount of weight, such as 10% over 6 months, can improve health for overweight and obese patients; losing weight slowly (1/2 to 2 pounds per week) is usually more effective for long-term weight management.
- To lose weight at this rate, the patient will need to consume 500 to 1000 kcal less per day than usual.

(Continued on following page)

- Assess the patient for physical signs of malnutrition and deficiency state as listed in Appendix P.
- Assess patient's salt intake. Be aware of hidden salt in canned goods and processed foods.
- Instruct patient in how to read nutrition labels.

Pediatric

- Explain goals of basic nutrition to parents.
- Explain introduction of foods to infant:
  - <u>0 to 4 months:</u> Breast milk or formula only.
  - <u>4 months:</u> Breast milk or formula. Cereal made with breast milk or formula should be fed with spoon. Begin with 1 teaspoon twice daily: Increase to 4 tablespoons twice daily.
  - <u>4 1/2 to 5 months:</u> Add vegetables one at a time. Give for 1 week before starting another. Begin with 1 teaspoon; increase to 3 tablespoons twice daily.
  - <u>5 months:</u> Add fruits one at a time, in same way you introduced vegetables.
  - <u>6 to 8 months:</u> Add meats, one meat at a time, for a week as you introduced vegetables and fruits. Add beef last. Add fruit juice diluted with half water.
  - Continue to give formula or breast milk for 1 year, then whole milk until age 2. After 2 years give 2% milk.
- Encourage parents to offer a wide variety of nutritious foods and to avoid offering foods containing empty calories such as soft drinks, candy, and pastries.
- Explain toddler-preschool eating patterns, that is, food jags or strong preference for only a few foods. Teach parents to assess diet over several days rather than over one meal.
- Discuss the need for fat in the infant's and toddler's diet.
- Explain hazards of choking when toddler eats hot dogs or hard candy or chews on toys or balloons.

Geriatric (See also App. Q)

- Teach techniques to prevent constipation:
  - Participate in regular exercise.

(Continued on following page)

Geriatric (See also App. Q) *(Continued)*

- Drink at least 1500 to 2000 ml of fluid per day, unless contraindicated by other health problems such as congestive heart disease or renal disease.
- The following types of drugs may contribute to constipation: antihistamines, aspirin, antacids with aluminum or calcium, antiparkinsonism drugs, diuretics, tranquilizers, and hypnotics.
- Reduce or eliminate use of laxatives because they can be harmful and habit forming.
- Eat foods high in fiber, such as fresh fruits and vegetables and whole grains. Eat foods low in fat and refined sugar.
- It is not necessary to have a bowel movement every day. Individuals have different patterns for elimination. If a person is not having problems with painful movements or hard stools and the frequency of movements is only once every 4 days or more, then the person is probably not constipated.
- Try to develop a regular schedule for bowel elimination, such as in the morning after breakfast.
- Respond promptly to the urge to defecate.
- Provide the following information to patients with fecal incontinence:
  - It is important to seek help and receive a comprehensive workup to determine the etiology.
  - Follow the same recommendations for fecal incontinence as those given above for constipation.
  - If fecal impaction or long-term constipation is the problem, initiate the above recommendations following removal of the impaction.
  - Establish a consistent toileting program and establish a routine time.
  - Instruct patient on pelvic muscle exercises.
  - Provide frequent reminders of the location of the restroom if the patient is cognitively impaired or in an unfamiliar environment.
  - Teach patient to be meticulous in skin care, use of absorbent products or external collection devices, and use of moisture barrier creams and to frequently assess the condition of the skin.

(Continued on following page)

Cultural

- Teach healthier variations in preparation of foods preferred in culture (e.g., boiled instead of fried, spices added to foods instead of salt).
- If lactose-intolerant (common in many Asians, African-Americans, Jews, and Mexican-Americans), suggest purchase of lactose-free milk or substitute other foods containing calcium such as yogurt.

Associated Community Agencies

- Food Stamp program: Serves all ages
- Supplemental Nutrition Program for Women, Infants, and Children (WIC): Serves pregnant and breast-feeding women and children up to the age of 5
- Reduced price and free lunches, school breakfast program: For school age children
- Congregate meal sites: Persons age 60 and older
- Meals on Wheels: Meals brought to home if no one in home is able to prepare
- Food pantries: At local churches or community centers (Contact United Way for information.)
- Ostomy clubs
- National Digestive Diseases Clearinghouse
- Celiac Sprue Association
- Crohn's and Colitis Foundation of America

CHAPTER **17**

Musculoskeletal System

 History

- Patient's age
- Last menstrual period or years since menopause
- Weight
- Height, loss of height
- Tobacco use
- Ability to care for self, functional abilities
- Exercise patterns, equipment: athletic injuries
- Knowledge and use of proper body mechanics, safety precautions
- <u>Muscular complaints:</u> Limitation of movement, weakness, tremor, tic, paralysis, clumsiness
- Assess dietary calcium, vitamin D, protein intake
- History of joint pain, swelling, heat, arthritis, bone injury (see App. R)
- <u>Skeletal complaints:</u> Difficulty with gait, limping, numbness, pain with movement, crepitus
- Joint, bone, muscle trauma
- Use of hormone replacement therapy
- <u>Medications:</u> Anti-inflammatory agents, aspirin
- Self or family history of osteoporosis, arthritis, fractures, muscle disease, tuberculosis, genetic or congenital disorders, cancer, scoliosis
- Orthopedic surgeries
- <u>Employment:</u> Possibility of fracture caused by injuries at work

Pediatric

Infant
- Birth injuries, macrosomia
- Alignment of hips, knees, ankles

(Continued on following page)

- Trauma
- Developmental milestones

Children

- Participation in sports, outdoor activities
- Frequent contact or high-impact fractures, limping, complaints of aches or pain in joints, other trauma
- Fractures at different stages of healing

Geriatric

- Stiffness, backache
- History of falls, tremors, spontaneous fractures, fall-related fractures, stumbling
- <u>Weakness or pain with muscle use:</u> Location; weakness and activity altered
- Problems with manual dexterity
- Deformity or coordination difficulties
- Problems with shoes
- Restless legs; transient paresthesia
- <u>Alterations in gait:</u> Weakness, balance problems, difficulty with steps, fear of falling
- <u>Use of assistive devices:</u> Walker, cane, grab bars, elevated toilet seat, wheelchair
- Joint swelling, pain, redness, heat, deformity, stiffness: Pronounced at certain times of day/night, or associated with or following activity or inactivity
- <u>Limited movement:</u> Specify.
- Crepitation
- Able to carry out ADLs and IADLs. If not, who is available for assistance?
- Assess for unexplained injuries such as bruises

Equipment

- Tape measure
- Goniometer

Patient Preparation

- Sitting
- Supine
- Standing (observation of balance)
- Walking (observation of gait)
- Observation of child while playing

Physical Assessment: Musculoskeletal System

Adult

Steps	Normal and/or Common Findings	Significant Deviations
Inspection		
• *Posture:* Note symmetry, erectness	Erect, flexible, mobile, slumped, rounded shoulders	Spinal curvatures (Fig. 17-1) Legs of uneven length
• *Major muscle groups:* Note symmetry	Atrophy, mild hypertrophy, bilateral symmetry	Marked or unexplained hypertrophy, asymmetry Marked or unexplained atrophy
• *Joints:* Note color; observe neck, shoulder, elbow, wrist, hip, knee, ankle, foot (Figs. 17-2 through 17-5)	Full ROM	Edema, redness, heat, limitation in motion, deformities
• *Spine:* Have patient bend at waist	Full ROM	Curvature Kyphosis (see Fig. 17-1) Scoliosis Lordosis
Palpation		
• *Joints:* Note mobility, range of motion (ROM) symmetry, temperature	Full active and passive ROM	Tenderness, warmth, edema, stiffness, instability
• *Muscles:* Note tone and strength by having patient resist pressure; compare bilaterally	Firm, tense on movement Strength 3+ to 4+	Soft, flabby Weakness 1+

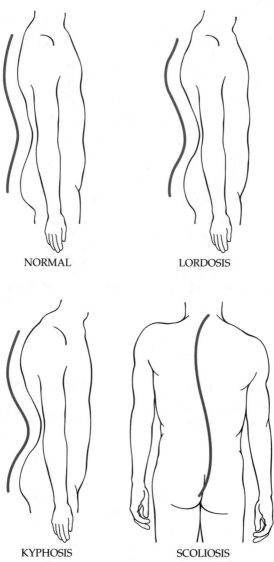

NORMAL   LORDOSIS

KYPHOSIS   SCOLIOSIS

Figure 17-1 Normal and abnormal spinal curves.

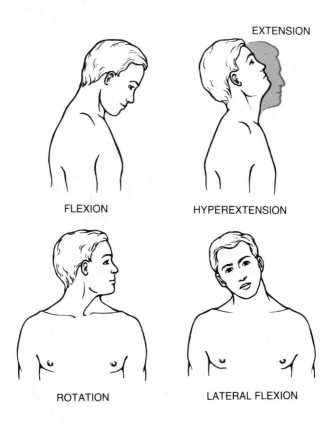

Figure 17-2 Range of motion of neck.

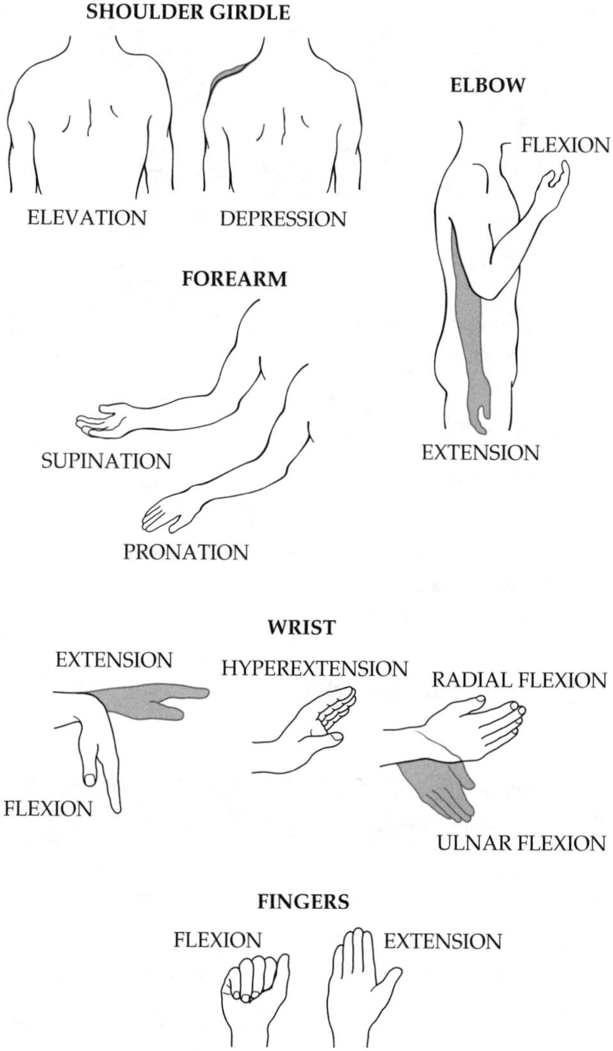

Figure 17-3 Range of motion of upper extremity.

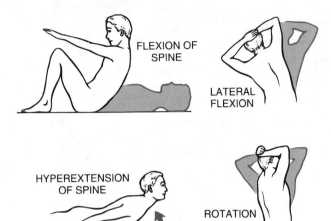

Figure 17-4 Range of motion of trunk.

Physical Assessment: Musculoskeletal System

Pediatric Adaptations

INFANT

Steps	Normal and/or Common Findings	Significant Deviations
Inspection • Muscle tone	Isotonic	Decreased muscle tone Hypertonic Scissoring
• *Feet, legs:* Note tibial torsion and/or metatarsus adductus; if present, use gentle pressure in attempt to straighten foot	Tibial torsion (should resolve after 6 months of age), flatfeet	Polydactyly or syndactyly Inability to straighten foot Clubfoot

(Continued on page 234)

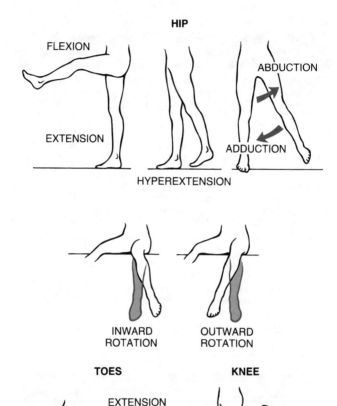

Figure 17-5 Range of motion of lower extremity.

(Continued)

Steps	Normal and/or Common Findings	Significant Deviations
Palpation		
• Clavicles	Intact	Fractures
• Hips	Equal gluteal folds, equal movement	Ortolani's sign (dislocation) (Fig. 17–6)
		Barlow's sign
		Unequal gluteal folds, limited ROM
• Spine	Intact, smooth	Defects in vertebral column, dimples, or hair tufts
• ROM	Full in all joints but may resist	
• *Muscles:* Note bilateral strength	May elicit Moro response	Hypertonicity, flaccidity, unilateral weakness

Physical Assessment: Musculoskeletal System

Pediatric Adaptations

CHILD

Steps	Normal and/or Common Findings	Significant Deviations
Inspection		
• Legs	Genu varum (bowleg) and metatarsus adductus (normal to age 2)	Asymmetry
		Toeing in
• Knees	Genu valgum (knock-knee) (from ages 2–10)	More than 2 1/2 in between malleolus when knees are touching
• Spine	Increased lumbar curvature in toddlers	Scoliosis

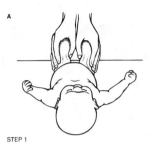

STEP 1

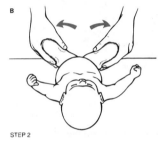

STEP 2

Figure 17-6 Hip dislocation in infant: Step 1: Flex infant's hips and knees. Place middle finger over greater trochanter. Step 2: Barlow-Ortolani maneuver—Abduct and adduct the thigh while in flexed position, feeling for a click or popping at greater trochanter.

Physical Assessment: Musculoskeletal System

Geriatric Adaptations

Steps	Normal and/or Common Findings	Significant Deviations
Inspection (Patient sitting)		
• Spine	Mild kyphosis	Severe kyphosis, scoliosis
• Joints of fingers, hands, wrists, shoulders, elbows, knees, ankles, toes	Limitation in normal ROM, instability	Swelling, nodules, heat, redness, crepitus, deformities (Fig. 17-7) Varus deformity (bowlegs) Valgus deformity (knock-knees)

(Continued on following page)

(Continued)

Steps	Normal and/or Common Findings	Significant Deviations
Inspection (*Continued*) • Muscles	Decreased muscle mass	Gross atrophy
• Feet	Corns, calluses, hammertoes, bunions	Joint swelling, redness
Test (Patient standing) • *Spine:* Note ROM, symmetry, posture	Abnormal curvature, especially kyphosis; slowed movement, diminished sense of balance; diminished muscle mass and strength bilaterally	Severe kyphosis, lordosis, scoliosis
Test (Patient sitting) • *ROM:* Check neck, fingers, hands, wrists, shoulders, elbows	Diminished joint flexibility bilaterally	ROM significantly impaired, affecting functional ability, marked pain
• *ROM:* Check ankles, feet, knees, hips	Diminished joint flexibility bilaterally	Joint swelling and redness
Palpation • Joint ROM		Crepitus, tenderness

Diagnostic Tests

May need to refer for:
• Bone densitometry to detect osteoporosis
• Blood tests for rheumatoid factor, calcium, and uric acid
• X-rays to detect compression fractures or other bone or joint abnormalities

Possible Nursing Diagnoses

• Injury, risk for
• Mobility, impaired physical
• Sleep pattern disturbance
• Protection, altered

- Activity intolerance, risk for
- Fatigue
- Self-care deficit, toilet
- Pain, chronic
- Disuse syndrome, risk for
- Social isolation

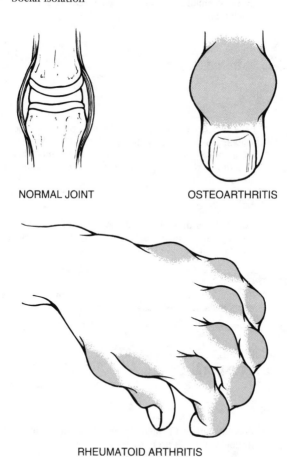

NORMAL JOINT   OSTEOARTHRITIS

RHEUMATOID ARTHRITIS

Figure 17-7 Normal joint and deformities.

Clinical Alert

- Protect older patients from falling.
- Prevent contractures by exercise and ROM activities.
- Refer if there is sudden joint pain, swelling, erythema or ROM limitation, sudden muscle weakness, or new back pain.

Sample Documentation

Adult

- Posture relaxed, erect; no lordosis, kyphosis, scoliosis visible. Joints mobile, nontender; full ROM demonstrated in every joint without pain or limitation. Muscle strength and size equal bilaterally. Gait smooth and steady.

Infant

- Extremities symmetrical, isotonic. Hips stable bilaterally. Spine straight, no tufts or dimples. Forefeet in varus position. Full passive ROM.

Child

- Extremities symmetrical, isotonic. Full ROM in all four extremities. No scoliosis.

Patient and Family Education and Home Health Notes

Adult

- Instruct patient to maintain muscle strength and joint flexibility through exercise.
- Teach appropriate exercise techniques.

(Continued on following page)

- Teach risk factors associated with osteoporosis (sedentary lifestyle, inadequate dietary calcium, female, small bones, low weight, white, fair skin, smoking, heavy caffeine or alcohol use). Encourage prevention beginning in youth, extending through lifetime.
- Teach safety risks associated with falls in home, such as multiple small stairs, loose rugs, poor lighting, uneven surfaces, wet surfaces (tub, bathroom floor).
- Instruct patient to have a physical exam before beginning exercise program.
  - Be physically active every day for at least 30 minutes. Some adults may need more physical activity to manage their weight.
  - Before exercise, stretch and warm up.
  - During exercise, maintain heart rate of between 60 and 85 percent of capacity. Calculate this by subtracting age from 220. Multiply this number by 0.60 to find the lower range and by 0.85 to obtain the higher range.
  - Cool down with stretching and milder exercise.

Pediatric

- Encourage physical fitness early with regular exercise.
- See Adult notes (above). Teach parents and adolescents about prevention of osteoporosis as well as maintenance of mobility.
- Teach safety precautions for the home.
- Instruct in use of protective devices when rollerblading and biking.

Geriatric

- Teach proper diet and exercise to reduce progression of osteoporosis.
- Teach about new methods to diagnose, treat, and reverse osteoporosis.

(Continued on following page)

- Teach patient how to manage chronic pain with pre-scribed medications and other modalities as appropriate (transcutaneous electrical nerve stimulation [TENS] unit, individualized exercise program, appropriate rest periods, articular rest, heat or cold therapy, paraffin baths for hands, splints or other assistive devices, weight loss, hydrotherapy and/or water exercises, surgical intervention).
- Teach patient how to use assistive devices correctly.
- Teach patient to avoid immobility.
- Risk factors:

  Environmental hazards—slippery or uneven walking surface, poor lighting, using stairs, throw rugs, small pets, bath tubs without grab handles, inappropriate footware (high heels, leather soles), rising from low chairs, changing position, and risk-taking behaviors

  Medications—analgesics—especially narcotics, psychotropics, antihypertensives, diuretics, and phenothiazines

  Physical—dementia, Parkinson's disease, stroke, peripheral neuropathy, cataracts, glaucoma, macular degeneration, arthritis, positional vertigo, foot disorders, muscle weakness, hypotension, and metabolic disease

- Teach safety measures to prevent falls:
  - Install nonslip mats and/or stick-ons in tubs and showers.
  - Use adequate lighting devices such as nonglare surfaces and night lights near stairs and/or stairwells.
  - Remove hazards such as throw rugs, electrical cords, loose carpet edges, clutter, and furniture from traffic pathways.
  - Hold onto rails along stairways for stabilization and support.
  - Ambulate with eyes facing ahead to scan the environment for any safety hazards.
  - Place grab bars near the toilet and tub.
  - Wear footwear with nonskid soles.
  - Ambulate carefully and do not rush.

(Continued on following page)

- Rise from a sitting position to a standing position very slowly to prevent orthostatic hypotension.
- Use emergency alert systems if they are available.
- If a patient is being seen in the home, assess and document his or her homebound status on each visit.
- When patients have decreased mobility:
  - Observe ambulation.
  - Instruct in use of assistive devices.
  - If walker or wheelchair is to be used, check width of hallways and doorways for maneuverability.
  - Check proximity of bathroom to bedroom.
  - Adjust height of walker, commode, and/or cane prn.
  - Instruct in use of hospital bed and the importance of turning.
  - Patient may need physical or occupational therapy evaluation and/or treatment to optimize function and safety.

Cultural

- Average Asian males are shorter than average white males.
- Average Asian females are shorter than average white females.
- Bones of average African-Americans are longer, larger, and denser than those of other groups and are less apt to fracture.
- Bone density is the least in Asians.

◼ Associated Community Agencies

- Arthritis Foundation: Arthritis self-help course, loans for equipment, public education
- American Red Cross: Transportation assistance
- Home health agencies: Homemaker assistance
- Churches: Help with building wheelchair ramps

- National Osteoporosis Foundation
- American Juvenile Arthritis Foundation
- Muscular Dystrophy Association
- National Scoliosis Foundation
- United Cerebral Palsy Association

CHAPTER **18**

Neurologic System

 History

Adult

- Headaches
- Dizziness
- Visual disturbances
- Numbness, weakness, spasms
- Twitching, tremors
- Forgetfulness
- History of head injury, neurosurgery, nerve injury, syncope, hereditary disorders such as Tay-Sachs disease, Huntington's disease, muscular dystrophy
- Changes in senses of taste, smell, hearing
- Difficulty swallowing
- Speech difficulties
- Seizures
- Change in cognition, behavior, communication, memory
- Use of all medications: Antidepressants, anticonvulsants, antivertigo agents
- Use of alcohol or mood-altering medications
- Exposure to chemicals, pesticides
- Exposure to assault (e.g., spousal abuse)
- History of cerebrovascular accident (CVA) in self or family

(Continued on following page)

Pediatric

Infant
- Apgar score of infant (see App. G)
- Birth trauma; other trauma or infection
- Maternal alcohol or substance abuse
- Maternal or neonatal exposure to TORCH viruses (Toxoplasmosis, Other [Syphilis], Rubella, Cytomegalovirus, Herpes Simplex)
- Dietary intake for 24 hours
- Patterns of behavior and daily schedule
- Child-rearing practices, risk of abuse

Child
- Past head injuries, illnesses, fevers
- Attainment of developmental milestones: Exhibits head control, sitting, crawling, walking, speaking, fine motor control
- Change in behavior, personality, cognition, communication
- Daily schedule, preschool, games
- Fever, projectile vomiting
- Amount and type of television viewed
- Interactions
- Use of drugs
- Neck stiffness, high-pitched cry
- Child-rearing practices, risk of abuse

Geriatric

- <u>Sensory disturbances:</u> Paresthesia, hyperesthesia, diplopia
- Dizziness, faintness, spells, attacks, weakness, headaches
- Changes in gait, coordination, and balance; vertigo
- History of injuries or falls, particularly recent ones
- Mental status changes such as in mood, thinking process, or cognitive process
- Speech alterations
- How any symptoms affect ADLs

Equipment

- Tuning fork
- Reflex hammer
- Cotton balls
- Familiar object: Coin, paper clip, button
- Sharp object

Patient Preparation

- Sitting
- Standing

Physical Assessment: Neurologic System

Adult

Steps	Normal and/or Common Findings	Significant Deviations
Motor/Sensory		
Inspection		
• *Extremities:* Note coordination, gait, tremor	Smooth motions, no tremor	Tremor; abnormal gaits such as shuffling
• *Large muscles:* Note symmetrical size, involuntary movements	No involuntary movement Symmetrical (Muscles of dominant side may be slightly larger)	
Test		
• *Romberg:* Have patient stand with both eyes open, then closed, with arms at sides, feet together (20–30 seconds) Stand near patient in case balance is lost	Minimal or no swaying	Drift, imbalance

(Continued on following page)

Steps	Normal and/or Common Findings	Significant Deviations
Palpation		
• *Extremities:* Note touch perception (with cotton ball), vibratory perception (with tuning fork over bone); distinguish between sharp and dull	Equal perception of vibration	Absent or asymmetrical vibratory perception
• *Large muscles:* Note symmetrical strength against resistance	Symmetrical	Unequal weakness
Reflexes		
Test		
• Biceps, triceps, brachioradialis, patellar knee jerk, Achilles, plantar (Figs. 18–1 through 18-3) using percussion hammer (Fig. 18-4)	+2	Diminished or increased responses
Cognition and/or Mental Status		
(See Apps. D, E, and A-K-9)		
Test		
• Orientation to person, place, time	Oriented × 3	Unable to orient self, setting, date
• *Memory:* Immediate, recent, remote, and old recall	Intact	Memory loss of significant immediate or recent events
• Affect and mood	Appropriate to setting and circumstance	Inappropriate emotional response
• Judgment and ability to abstract	Responds appropriately	Judgment impaired
• Thought content and process		Inappropriate
Cranial Nerves		
(Table 18-1)		
Test		
(If not tested with above systems)		

(Continued on page 249)

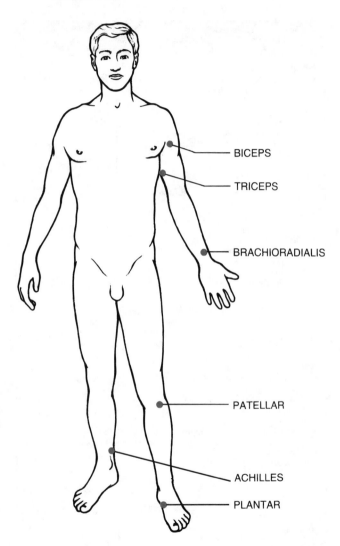

Figure 18-1 Reflexes.

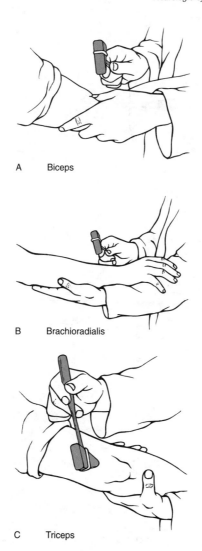

A   Biceps

B   Brachioradialis

C   Triceps

Figure 18-2 Eliciting deep tendon reflexes.

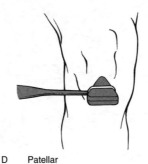

D   Patellar

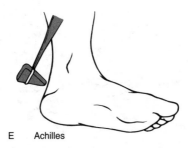

E   Achilles

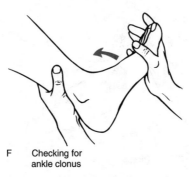

F   Checking for
ankle clonus

Figure 18-2 *(Continued)* Eliciting deep tendon reflexes.

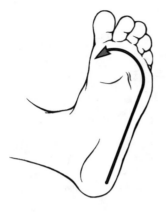

Figure 18-3 Eliciting deep tendon reflexes.

(Continued)

Steps	Normal and/or Common Findings	Significant Deviations
Test (Continued)		
• *CN I:* Ability to identify odors	Able to identify specific odors	Absence of sense of smell
• *CN II:* Visual acuity	Able to visualize all fields	
• *CN III:* Pupils, extraocular movements (EOMs)	Pupils constrict, eyes move through fields symmetrically	Asymmetrical pupillary response
• *CN IV:* Lid movements, EOMs	Even and symmetrical lid and eye movements	Nystagmus
• *CN V:* Facial sensation, muscle strength, corneal reflexes	Equal sensation and strength	Decreased or absent sensation; absent or asymmetrical blink
• *CN VI:* Lateral eye movements	Blink symmetrical EOMs	Absent or asymmetrical lateral eye movements
• *CN VII:* Facial muscle strength, taste	Symmetrical strength	Dropping lid Paralysis Decreased strength
• *CN VIII:* Hearing acuity, sound conduction	Equal acuity	Hearing loss
• *CN IX:* Taste, gag reflex	Voice smooth, gag reflex intact	Hoarseness; soft palate fails to rise or uvula deviates laterally

(Continued on following page)

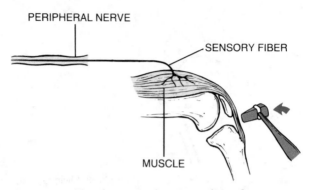

Figure 18-4 Use of percussion hammer to elicit reflex response.

(Continued)

Steps	Normal and/or Common Findings	Significant Deviations
Test *(Continued)*		
• *CN X:* Symmetry of uvula movement	Symmetrical rising of soft palate	Asymmetrical or diminished movement
• *CN XI:* Neck and shoulder strength	Symmetrical strength of trapezii and sternocleidomastoid muscles	Weakness, unilateral or bilateral
• *CN XII:* Tongue: control, symmetry, strength	Even strength and motion of tongue	Fasciculations or deviation of tongue

Table 18-1

Cranial Nerve Functions and Assessment Methods

Cranial Nerve	Name	Type	Function	Assessment Methods
I	Olfactory	Sensory	Smell	Ask patient to close eyes and identify different mild aromas, such as coffee, tobacco, vanilla, oil of cloves, peanut butter, orange, lemon, lime, chocolate.
II	Optic	Sensory	Vision and visual fields	Ask patient to read Snellen chart; check visual fields by confrontation, and conduct an ophthalmoscopic examination.
III	Oculomotor	Motor	Extraocular movement (EOM); movement of sphincter of pupil; movement of ciliary muscles of lens	Assess six ocular movements and pupil reactions.
IV	Trochlear	Motor	EOM, specifically moves eyeball downward and laterally	Assess six ocular movements.

(Continued on following page)

Table 18-1 *(Continued)*

Cranial Nerve Functions and Assessment Methods

Cranial Nerve	Name	Type	Function	Assessment Methods
V	Trigeminal Ophthalmic branch	Sensory	Sensation of cornea, skin of face, and nasal mucosa	While patient looks upward, lightly touch lateral sclera of eye to elicit blink reflex. To test light sensation, have patient close eyes; then wipe a wisp of cotton over patient's forehead and paranasal sinuses. To test deep sensation, alternately use blunt and sharp ends of a safety pin over same areas.
	Maxillary branch	Sensory	Sensation of skin of face and anterior oral cavity (tongue and teeth)	Assess skin sensation as for ophthalmic branch above.
	Mandibular branch	Motor and sensory	Muscles of mastication; sensation of skin of face	Ask patient to clench teeth.
VI	Abducens	Motor	EOM; moves eyeball laterally	Assess six cardinal fields of gaze.
VII	Facial	Motor and sensory	Facial expression; taste (anterior two-thirds of tongue)	Ask patient to smile, raise the eyebrows, frown, puff out cheeks, close eyes tightly. Ask patient to identify

various tastes placed on tip and sides of tongue; sugar (sweet), salt, lemon juice (sour), and quinine (bitter). Identify areas of taste.

VIII	Auditory Vestibular branch	Sensory	Equilibrium	Assessment methods are discussed with cerebellar functions (in next section).
	Cochlear branch	Sensory	Hearing	Assess patient's ability to hear spoken word and vibrations of tuning fork.
IX	Glossopharyngeal	Motor and sensory	Swallowing ability and gag reflex, tongue movement, taste (posterior tongue)	Use tongue blade on posterior tongue while patient says "ah" to elicit gag reflex. Apply tastes on posterior tongue for identification. Ask patient to move tongue from side to side and up and down.
X	Vagus	Motor and sensory	Sensation of pharynx and larynx; swallowing; vocal cord movement	Assessed with CN IX; assess patient's speech for hoarseness.
XI	Accessory	Motor	Head movement; shrugging of shoulders	Ask patient to shrug shoulders against resistance from your hands and turn head to side against resistance from your hand. Repeat for other side.
XII	Hypoglossal	Motor	Protrusion of tongue	Ask patient to protrude tongue at midline; then move it side to side.

Source: *From Kozier, B; Erb, G, Berman, A, and Snyder, S: Fundamentals of Nursing, ed 7, p. 614. Copyright 2004 by Pearson Prentice Hall. Reprinted by permission.*

📕 Physical Assessment: Neurologic System

Pediatric Adaptations

INFANT

Steps	Normal and/or Common Findings	Significant Deviations
Inspection		
• *Behavior:* Note alertness, positioning	Irritability	Extreme irritability, tremors Brudzinski's or Kernig's sign
• *Crying:* Note pitch of cry		High-pitched or cat's cry
• *Reflexes:* Moro, tonic neck, palmar and plantar grasp, Babinski, rooting, sucking	All present in term newborn	Absence of reflexes
• Neck righting	4-6 months old	
• Parachute	8-9 months old	
• Muscle tone	Firm recoil	Flaccid
• Observe for appropriate parent-infant interactions, stranger anxiety, parent's ability to soothe infant	Separation anxiety greatest at 8-20 months	Inappropriate interactions and parental expectations; no separation anxiety
Palpation		
• Anterior and posterior fontanels	Soft and flat	Bulging or markedly depressed
• *Touch:* Note response to touch in extremities in quiet-alert state	Moves to touch	No response; exaggerated, jerky response; asymmetrical response
Test		
• *Hearing:* Note acoustic activity	Responds by waking, or turning toward sound, or movement	No response to sounds
• Pupils	Pupils equal, round, and reactive to light and accommodation (PERRLA)	Unequal pupillary response

(Continued on following page)

Steps	Normal and/or Common Findings	Significant Deviations
Cranial Nerves		
• CN II, III, IV, VI	Infant should blink when light is shined in eyes	Absent, asymmetrical, or diminished response for each area tested for nerves I through XI
• CN V	Rooting and sucking reflex present	
• CN VII	Facial symmetry when crying, sucking, rooting	
• CN VIII	Blink or Moro reflex in response to clapping near side of head	
• *CN I and XI:* Cannot be tested in the infant		
• *CN IX and X:* Similar to the adult		

Physical Assessment: Neurologic System

Pediatric Adaptations

CHILD

Steps	Normal and/or Common Findings	Significant Deviations
Inspection		
• Observe for appropriate parent-child interaction	Increasing independence of child, decreasing control by parent	Communication unclear; hostility; aggression; dependence
• *Cerebral dominance:* Observe child while at play	Preference for one hand or the other usually evident by age 3–4	
Test		
• Speech	3-year-olds should be able to speak so that others can understand them 90% of the time	Unclear speech

(Continued on following page)

(Continued)

Steps	Normal and/or Common Findings	Significant Deviations
Cranial Nerves • *CN II:* Snellen eye chart with pictures or E chart • *CN III, IV, VI:* Use a new toy to test cardinal positions • *CN V:* May offer child a cracker to test muscular strength of jaw • Remaining CNs may be tested as for an adult • Children who are 3–6 years old should be evaluated by the Denver II		Abnormal results on the Denver II

🔲 Physical Assessment: Neurologic System

Geriatric Adaptations

Steps	Normal and/or Common Findings	Significant Deviations
Inspection • Face		Tremors, asymmetry such as drooping of side of mouth, drooling from one side of mouth, asymmetrical wrinkling of forehead **or subtle asymmetry of lines at corners of mouth**
• Extremities		Tremors, unilateral or symmetrical weakness, gait disturbances
• Emotional responses		Labile, severely agitated, major behavioral changes

(Continued on following page)

Steps	Normal and/or Common Findings	Significant Deviations
Test		
• *Mental acuity:* Note alterations	Diminished memory for recent events	Marked change in mental status, poor judgment, limited attention span
• Heel-to-shin movement	May not be able to perform	
• Gait	Decreased balance, muscle tone, short steps, wide stance, slower gait	Gross unsteadiness, rigid arm movements, shuffling, marked impairment in balance and/or stability, extreme wide-based gait
• *Equilibrium:* Note: Do not ask geriatric patients to perform deep knee bends or hop in place on one foot; most normal older people cannot do these maneuvers because of impaired position sense. Instead, observe patient rising from chair	Diminished; decreased vibratory sense in toes	Severe swaying, unable to maintain balance, absent vibratory sensation in lower extremities
Percussion		
• Deep tendon reflexes	May be diminished, especially the Achilles reflex	Hyperactive, absent, asymmetrical
Cranial Nerves		
• CN I	Sense of smell diminished	See significant deviations for the adult; sense of smell absent
• CN II	Presbyopia corrected with glasses	Marked loss of vision Diminished peripheral vision Diminished color discrimination (especially blues, greens, and purples)
• CN III	Pupil size diminished, impaired accommodation, diminished upward gaze	Nonreactive pupils

(Continued on following page)

(Continued)

Steps	Normal and/or Common Findings	Significant Deviations
Cranial Nerves *(Continued)*		
• CN V	Sensory perception of pain; light touch may be diminished	Absent
• CN VII	Diminished sense of taste	Absent
• CN VIII	Diminished hearing, especially of high-frequency sounds	Significant hearing loss
• CN IX and X	Diminished taste perception on posterior tongue	Absent
• CN XI	Diminished muscle strength	Marked muscle weakness, interferes with ADLs

🔖 Diagnostic Tests

May need to refer for:
* CT scan
* MRI
* EEG
* Electrolytes, CBC, sedimentation rate, thyroid function tests, vitamin B_{12} and folate levels, rapid plasma reagin (RPR)
* Spinal tap
* Neuropsychiatric testing

🔖 Possible Nursing Diagnoses

* Communication, impaired verbal
* Coping, individual, ineffective
* Mobility, impaired physical
* Swallowing, impaired
* Sensory perceptual alterations (specify): Visual, auditory, kinesthetic, gustatory, tactile, olfactory
* Thought processes, altered
* Injury, risk for

Clinical Alert

- Differentiate symptoms of dementia, delirium, and depression, and refer all cognitive and behavioral changes for diagnosis and treatment.

📘 Sample Documentation

Adult

- Gait, coordination smooth and steady. Extremities symmetrically strong; touch and vibratory sense intact. Deep tendon reflexes (DTRs) symmetrically +2 (biceps, triceps, brachioradialis, knee-jerk, ankle). Oriented × 3: Immediate, recent, and remote memory intact: thought, emotion grossly appropriate. Cranial nerves I-XII intact. Babinski negative laterally. Fine motor coordination intact. Balance intact. Romberg negative. Speech clear and follows directions without difficulty.

Infant

- Alert. Fontanelle soft and flat. Moro and palmar grasp reflexes present. Positive Babinski. Normocephalic. PERRLA.

Child

- Alert, cooperative. Oriented × 3. Cranial nerves II-VIII intact. Climbs stairs unassisted. Denver II scores normal. PERRLA.

⬛ Patient and Family Education and Home Health Notes

Adult

- Prevent head injury with seat belts, helmets.
- Prevent motor vehicle accidents. Observe speed limits and do not drink and drive.
- Read labels of pesticides and chemicals, and observe precautions at home.
- Be aware of available information and services to deter violence, practice stress management, and do not abuse drugs.
- Follow ergonomic guidelines and safety practices at workplace and at home

Pediatric

- Discuss developmentally appropriate infant stimulation activities.
- Protect infants and toddlers from traumatic falls.
- Teach parents and children use of seat belts, helmets, and car seats.
- Encourage parents to make sure their children learn how to swim.
- Teach sports and recreation safety (e.g., use spotters for gymnastics, never swim alone, never dive in unknown waters, and observe cautions on toys, including age appropriateness).
- Teach parents how to avoid children's accidental ingestion of poisons, drugs, chemicals. All such products should be stored out of sight and reach, behind a locked door if possible.
- Instruct parents to post national poison control number on telephone: 1-800-222-1222. *(Continued on following page)*

Geriatric

- Maintain activities that stimulate the mind.
- Have diminished vision and hearing assessed and treated.
- Maintain physical activities and exercise.
- Take care to avoid extreme heat and cold.
- Use assistive devices correctly, and follow safety precautions for the sensory impaired. Prevent falls.
- Seek medical help immediately if mental status or marked behavioral changes are noted.

Associated Community Agencies

- National Spinal Cord Injury Association
- Alzheimer's Disease and Related Disorders Association
- Local chapter of the Mental Health Association
- Epilepsy Foundation of America
- Spina Bifida Association of America

CHAPTER **19**

Male Genitourinary System and Rectum

History

Adult

- Patient's age
- Diet, use of alcohol
- Frequency, urgency, dysuria, nocturia
- Difficulty starting or stopping urinary stream

(Continued on following page)

Adult   *(Continued)*

- Dribbling or weak stream
- Blood in urine; discharge
- Changes in bowel or bladder function
- Pain, lesions, or masses on penis, scrotum, inguinal area, anus
- Circumcised
- Back pain
- Contraceptive use
- Swelling of scrotum
- History of prostatitis UTIs, pyelonephritis, cancer, diabetes, arthritis, cardiac or respiratory disease
- History of surgery, trauma, hernia
- Infertility
- Satisfied with sexual activity
- Impotence, difficulty getting or maintaining erection, difficulty with ejaculation
- Sexually transmitted diseases (STDs)
- Self-examination techniques, frequency
- Sexual partner preference
- Risk factors for human immunodeficiency virus (HIV), safer sex practices
- Hemorrhoids
- Rectal bleeding, blood in stools, pain
- Use of protective or supportive devices when exercising
- Travel history, areas with high incidences of parasitic infection
- Family history of colon or prostate cancer, rectal polyps

Pediatric

- Number of wet diapers per day
- Perianal itching
- Meconium ileus
- Chronic constipation, diarrhea, mucorrhea, steatorrhea
- Enuresis
- Encopresis

(Continued on following page)

- UTIs
- Age of toilet training
- Congenital anomalies
- Hygiene practices: Circumcised, uncircumcised
- Scrotal swelling
- Mother's use of hormones during pregnancy
- Sexual activity (adolescent); knowledge level

Geriatric

- Duration and characteristics of urinary incontinence
- Frequency and amount of continent and incontinent voids
- Precipitants of incontinence
- Past treatments for urinary incontinence and its effects
- History of recurrent UTIs
- Other lower urinary tract symptoms: Frequency, urgency, dysuria, feeling of incomplete emptying or retention, straining to void, hesitancy in starting urine stream, weak urine stream, nocturia, hematuria, postvoid drip
- Use of condoms, catheters, briefs, or other protective products
- History of bowel habits: Constipation, fecal incontinence, or loose stools
- Fluid and dietary intake patterns
- Medications: Prescribed and OTC
- Urethral discharge or burning
- Functional or cognitive deficits that interfere with sexual activity or continence
- Decline in frequency of or satisfaction with sexual activity
- Any treatment or surgery for prostate enlargement or a hernia
- Erectile dysfunction (difficulty achieving or maintaining an erection sufficient for intercourse) or difficulties in achieving an orgasm
- Difficulty retracting the foreskin
- Anal sphincter tone

▦ Equipment

* Gloves
* Lubricant
* Thermometer (for neonates)
* Drapes
* Penlight

▦ Patient Preparation

* Supine
* Standing
* Bending over
* Consider developmental age in discussing exam with child

▦ Physical Assessment: Male Genitourinary System and Rectum

Adult

Steps	Normal and/or Common Findings	Significant Deviations
Inspection		
• *Hair:* Note distribution, foreign bodies	Parasites	
• Skin of penis, scrotum, inguinal area	Intact, smooth, wrinkled, rugae on scrotum	Lesions, rashes, nodules, edema, body lice
• *Penis:* Note prepuce, glans, foreskin, circumcision, position of urinary meatus (Table 19–1)	No lesions, discharge Foreskin easily retracted, if present Located at tip	Phimosis, chancre, warts, ulcers, discharge Displacement of meatus on dorsal or ventral side of penis
• Anus	Hemorrhoids	Lesions, polyps, bleeding Very tender or painful

(Continued on following page)

Table 19-1

Stages of Secondary Characteristics: Male Genital Development

Development	Characteristic
A. Hair growth	1. None
	2. Scant fine hair at the base of the penis
	3. Darker and curlier hair
	4. Adult type but less hair
	5. Adult
B. Genital development	1. No change
	2. Larger scrotum and testes, skin redder
	3. Enlargement of penis
	4. Further enlargement of penis, scrotal skin thickening
	5. Adult

Source: Data from Tanner, JM: Foetus into Man: Physical Growth From Conception to Maturity. Harvard University Press, Cambridge, Mass., 1990.

Steps	Normal and/or Common Findings	Significant Deviations
Palpation Use gloves		
• Shaft of penis	Slightly tender	Discharge from urinary meatus; nodules, masses, lesions
• *Testicles:* Note size	Smooth, one side usually larger than other, left side lower than right, freely movable; determine consistency—fluidfilled, gas, or solid material	Tenderness, nodules, ulcers, lesions, pain, enlarged
• Transluminate scrotum if mass other than testes		
• Inguinal, femoral area	No masses, nodes	Hernias, enlarged nodes
• Anus and rectum	Hemorrhoids	Inflammation, rashes, lesions, tenderness, induration Masses
• *Prostate:* With patient leaning over table, gently insert gloved, lubricated index finger into rectum; note size, consistency	Smooth, rubbery; should be able to palpate only about 1 cm of gland; soft	Tenderness, nodules, masses; >1 cm protruding into rectum; firm, hard

Physical Assessment: Male Genitourinary System and Rectum

Pediatric Adaptations

INFANT

Steps	Normal and/or Common Findings	Significant Deviations
Inspection		
• *Penis:* Note prepuce and glans	Smooth, nontender, moist; prepuce covers glans	Redness, tenderness, swelling
• *Urethral meatus:* Note placement; retract foreskin in uncircumcised males only enough to see urinary meatus; do not break adhesions	Centered at tip of penis	Hypospadias (meatus on ventral surface) Epispadias (meatus on dorsal surface)
• Scrotum	Well rugated	Absence of rugae or underdeveloped scrotum
• Anus	Patent	Absent, occluded, signs of trauma
• Meconium	Should pass within 24 hours of birth	Meconium ileus
Palpation		
• *Testicles:* To check for their presence in scrotum, position child crosslegged and sitting to prevent retraction of testes	Both palpable	Either or both absent
• Inguinal canal	Intact	Herniations, bulges
• *Test:* If perianal itching, place tape against perianal folds; examine with microscope	No nematodes visible	Nematodes Pinworms
• *Test:* Anal patency can be checked in neonates by cautiously inserting a lubricated rectal thermometer if stools are not passed within first 24 hours of life	Anus patent	Unable to insert thermometer

■ Physical Assessment: Male Genitourinary System and Rectum

Geriatric Adaptations

Steps	Normal and/or Common Findings	Significant Deviations
Inspection		
• *Pubic hair:* Note amount and distribution	Diminished if not absent	
• *Penis:* Retract foreskin, if present, to examine head of penis; note hygiene	Decreased in size Many men > age 75 have not been circumcised.	Drainage, infection, lesions, nodules, tenderness, swelling of penis, inability to retract foreskin, painful retraction
• Scrotum	Pendulous	Rashes, excoriation, lesions, edema, fewer rugae
Palpation		
• *Testes:* Note size	Small, atrophied	Enlarged, nodular, fixed, tender
• Rectum		Bleeding
• Prostate	Enlarged prostate, relaxed rectal sphincter tone	Fecal impaction, grossly lax sphincter tone, hemorrhoids, masses
		Markedly enlarged, boggy or rubbery, hard and nodular, tender

■ Diagnostic Tests

May need to refer for:

- Culture, if drainage is present
- Fecal swab for guaiac test
- Prostate-specific antigen (PSA), blood test, or prostate ultrasound or biopsy
- Urinalysis
- Urodynamic testing; comprehensive workup for urinary and/or fecal incontinence
- Sexual dysfunction workup

📘 Possible Nursing Diagnoses

- Infection, risk for
- Constipation
- Nutrition: altered, less than, more than
- Fluid volume deficit, risk for
- Urinary elimination, altered patterns of
- Urinary retention (acute/chronic)
- Sexual dysfunction
- Sexuality pattern, altered
- Self-care deficit, bathing/hygiene
- Self-care deficit, toilet
- Rape-trauma syndrome

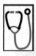

Clinical Alert

- Maintain patient's privacy and reduce embarrassment as much as possible.
- Prevent trauma to hemorrhoids.
- Refer any complaints of dysuria, hematuria, difficulty voiding, penile lesions, discharge, or sexual dysfunction

📘 Sample Documentation

Adult

- Skin of genitalia smooth, dry, nontender. Circumcised penis without discharge or lesions. Testes smooth, not enlarged. No hernias palpated. Prostate border palpable: smooth, firm, nontender. Rectum without internal or external hemorrhoids or masses. Small amount of soft stool palpable in lower rectal vault and sphincter tone strong. Perianal area intact: sphincter tightens evenly.

(Continued on following page)

- Penis uncircumcised. Foreskin retracts freely. Meatus at tip of penis. Testes descended bilaterally. Anus patent.

Patient and Family Education and Home Health Notes

- Instruct men to have rectal examination annually after age 40.
- Instruct male patients to begin testicular self-examination (TSE) (Fig. 19–1) in their midteens.
- Explain risks of STDs.
- Teach HIV Prevention
  - People become infected with HIV by having oral, anal or vaginal sex with someone who has HIV.
  - If sexually active, have oral, anal, or vaginal intercourse only with one mutually monogamous partner who does not use injection drugs and who is not infected with HIV.
  - Emphasize risks of having multiple sex partners.
  - Learn to correctly use latex barrier protection, like condoms, each and every time having oral, anal, or vaginal intercourse.
  - Do not have sex with multiple partners, with persons who have multiple partners, with persons who use injected drugs, or with persons who have or are at risk for having HIV infection.
  - Do not use drugs that can affect judgment, resulting in unsafe sex.
  - Do not share needles. This includes needles used for injecting drugs, vitamins, or steroids and needles used for tattooing and body piercing. Do not share the equipment or "works" for preparing injected drugs.
  - Do not share razors or toothbrushes.
  - Those who have had unprotected sex or shared needles with anyone should have an HIV test.

(Continued on following page)

Pediatric

- Explain testicular examination.
- Discuss sexual development and activities as appropriate for age.
- Teach parents and child how to keep uncircumcised penis clean.
- Discuss with parents ways to teach child to prevent sexual abuse.

Geriatric

- Encourage intake of 2000 to 3000 mL of fluid daily unless clinically contraindicated.
- Teach patient to avoid micturition syncope in bathroom as it could result in a serious fall. Teach patient to sit down to void.
- Following a transurethral resection of prostate (TURP), it is important that the patient understand that he will experience retrograde ejaculation.
- Sexual activity can continue well into a man's 90s or beyond, barring any major physical obstacles. Teach that it may take longer for an erection to occur, the erection may not be as firm as when he was younger, and it also may take more direct stimulation to achieve an erection. Ask physician about medications or devices if needed.
- If not circumcised, teach patient to keep head of penis clean.
- Teach male and female patient to use water-soluble lubricant if needed during intercourse.
- Fecal and urinary incontinence are treatable conditions, but it is crucial that the patient seek help from a healthcare provider early. If the healthcare provider does not respond to requests for testing and assistance with an incontinence problem, instruct patient to seek help from a specialist, such as a urologist, a geriatrician, or an advanced practice nurse who specializes in such problems.

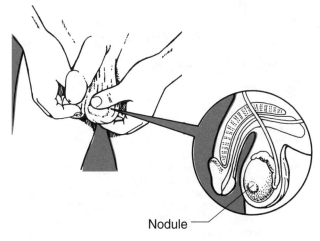

Nodule

Figure 19-1 Testicular self-examination. Instruct patient to roll each testicle gently between thumb and fingers of both hands, feeling for lumps or nodules.

◗ Associated Community Agencies

- National Association for Continence: Patient advocacy and education
- National Kidney Foundation: Local screening programs, education, and counseling
- National Kidney and Urologic Diseases Information Clearinghouse: Education
- Children's Organ Transplant Association
- Polycystic Kidney Disease Research Foundation

CHAPTER **20**

Female Genitourinary System and Rectum

History

- Menstrual history
  - Age at menarche
  - Last menstrual period
  - Character, length, regularity of menses
  - <u>Dysmenorrhea:</u> Nature, severity, treatment
  - <u>Premenstrual changes:</u> Nature, severity, treatment
- Sexual history
  - Age of first coital experience
  - Number of different partners
  - Sexual partner preference
  - Satisfactions, problems
- Contraceptive history
  - Current and previous methods used
  - <u>Current method:</u> Satisfaction, consistency, questions or problems noted
- Obstetric history
  - <u>Gravidity, parity:</u> Term, preterm, living children
  - <u>Abortions:</u> Spontaneous, induced
  - <u>Previous pregnancies:</u> Complications with pregnancy, delivery, newborn
- <u>Use of these products:</u> Douche, sprays, deodorants, antiseptic soaps, talcum powder
- Dates of last Pap smear and pelvic examination
- History of vaginitis, cystitis, pyelonephritis, in utero exposure to diethylstilbestrol (DES), STDs
- <u>Recent change in any of the following:</u> Bleeding, pain, vaginal discharge
- History of gynecologic/urologic surgeries
- History of sexual assault, incest; stage in crisis resolution
- Risk factors for HIV, safer sex practices

(Continued on following page)

- Urinary function:
  - Dysuria
  - Urinary urgency, frequency
  - Hematuria
  - Urinary incontinence
  - Infections: Chronic, related to coitus

Pediatric

- Hygenic practices:
  - Use of bubble baths, irritating soaps, powders
  - Number of layers of clothing
  - Wearing cotton underpants
  - Cleansing perineal area front to back
  - <u>Signs of sexual abuse:</u> Trauma, skin color changes in perineal area; history of bleeding, itching; inappropriate adultlike sexual knowledge, language, or behavior; sexually transmitted diseases

Geriatric

- Duration and characteristics of urinary incontinence
- Frequency and amount of continent and incontinent voids
- Precipitants of incontinence
- Past treatments for urinary incontinence and its effects
- History of recurrent UTIs
- <u>Other lower urinary tract symptoms:</u> Frequency, urgency, dysuria, feeling of incomplete emptying or retention, straining to void, hesitancy, nocturia, hematuria
- Use of pads, briefs, or other protective products
- History of constipation or loose stools
- Fluid and dietary intake patterns
- <u>Medications:</u> Prescribed and OTC
- Urethral and/or vaginal discharge or burning
- Functional or cognitive deficits that interfere with sexual activity or continence: any adaptations made
- <u>Reproductive history:</u> Number of children, types of deliveries, complications
- <u>Menopausal history:</u> Date, difficulties, satisfactions

(Continued on following page)

> Geriatric   *(Continued)*

- Soreness, tenderness, dryness of vaginal wall
- Dyspareunia: decline in frequency of or enjoyment of sexual activity caused by pain in the labia, vagina, or pelvis
- Pressure or heavy sensation in genital or pelvic area
- Vaginal bleeding after menopause
- Anal sphincter tone

Equipment

- Gown, drape
- New, clean glove
- Water-soluble lubricant
- Flexible floor lamp
- Pap smear equipment
- Speculum (may need pediatric size for both young women and older women who are no longer sexually active)
- Sterile cotton swabs/glass slide
- DNA probe kit for gonorrhea and *Chlamydia*

Patient Preparation

- Have patient empty bladder before examination.
- Drape fully in lithotomy position.
- Alternative positions may be necessary for women with disabilities.
- Offer mirror to explain findings to patient.
- Warm speculum to body temperature.
- Place child in frog-leg position.

Physical Assessment: External Structures

Adult

Steps	Normal and/or Common Findings	Significant Deviations
Inspection		
• *Hair:* Note distribution, amount, foreign bodies	Coarse, full, symmetrical	Uneven or unusually sparse Lice
• *Labia:* Note color, vascularity, moisture, symmetry, discharge, lesions, odor	Pink to red; moist, symmetrical Scant to moderate white, nonodorous discharge	Pale, inflamed Varicosities Dry Edema or swelling, especially unilaterally Dry, caked discharge Copious, watery, thickened, or foul-smelling, white-yellow or green discharge, lesions
• *Clitoris:* Note size, color, lesions	2×0.5 cm; same color as surrounding tissue	Atrophied or enlarged; reddened
• *Vaginal and urinary orifices:* Note color, lesions, moisture, size, bulging of vaginal wall	Pink to red, moist, smooth; no lesions bulging	Reddened; lesions (ulcers, blisters, condylomata acuminata), edematous irritated Bulging of anterior or posterior vaginal wall on straining
• *Anus:* Note integrity	Wrinkled, coarsened texture	Fissures, hemorrhoids (Fig. 20-1), lesions
Palpation		
• *Labia:* Note masses, tenderness, integrity	Smooth, nontender, homogeneous tissue	Nodules, painful to touch, irregularities
• *Skene glands:* Use one finger to press upward and laterally inside vagina, drawing finger toward outside of vagina; observe for drainage from gland	No discharge Openings not visible	Discharge (culture) Openings visible
• Bartholin glands	No tenderness or edema	Redness, tenderness, swelling of labia, especially unilaterally

(Continued on following page)

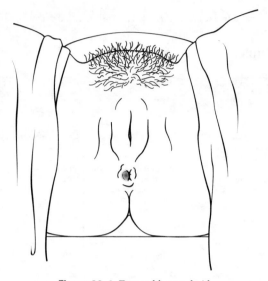

Figure 20-1 External hemorrhoid.

(Continued)

Steps	Normal and/or Common Findings	Significant Deviations
Palpation (Continued) • *Vaginal orifices:* Use thumb and forefinger; gently pinch around sides and perianal area; note tenderness, masses	No masses, non-tender	Nodules, painful to touch
• With finger in vagina, ask client to tighten muscles and bear down; note strength, bulges, urinary incontinence	Tight muscles, no bulges, no incontinence	Bulging of anterior or posterior wall, urinary incontinence, protrusion of cervix

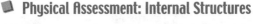 **Physical Assessment: Internal Structures**

Adult

To insert vaginal speculum: Warm speculum with water. Insert two fingers into vagina and press down firmly; insert closed speculum at an angle over fingers, keeping blades at 45-degree downward angle. Rotate speculum back to horizontal level and gently open blades.

Steps	Normal and/or Common Findings	Significant Deviations
Inspection		
• *Mucosa:* Note color, integrity, lesions, discharge	Pink to red; smooth, moist, clear to white odorless discharge	Bright red or pale; lesions, fissures, inflamed areas, discharge
• *Cervix:* Note color, position, surface, discharge, os, lesions	Evenly pink, midline, smooth surface or small, raised, light nabothian cysts Discharge odorless, clear to white; os small, round, or horizontal slit	Blue, reddened, pale Deviate laterally Patches of red or white tissue, friability increased Heavy, malodorous, yellow to green to gray discharge

Physical Assessment: Obtaining Pap Smears

Adult

With speculum in place, obtain cells from cervical os, cervical border, and vaginal pool. Use spatula and cytobrush, and label slides with client's name and birth date before spraying with fixative. (To withdraw speculum: Close blades, rotate 45 degrees, gently remove, and avoid pinching.)

Steps	Normal and/or Common Findings	Significant Deviations
Palpation Insert gloved index and middle fingers into vagina and place nondominant hand on lower abdomen; trap internal structures between your hands		

(Continued on following page)

(Continued)

Steps	Normal and/or Common Findings	Significant Deviations
Palpation (Continued)		
• *Cervix:* Note consistency, surface, position, mobility, tenderness, patency of os	Firm, smooth, midline, mobile to 2 cm, nontender, patent	Boggy, nodules, lateral deviations, fixed, painful with lateral movement, strictures at os
• *Uterus:* Note position, size, shape, mobility, tenderness, masses	Midline; pearshaped, 6–8 cm in length, slight AP mobility without tenderness	Lateral deviation, unilateral or bilateral masses, fixed, tender or painful to touch
• *Ovaries:* Note size, shape, tenderness, consistency, masses	May not be palpable; approximately 3 × 2 cm, slightly tender, smooth, firm	Enlarged, nodular, asymmetrical, painful
Change gloves. Lubricate; insert index finger into vagina, middle finger into rectum		
• *Uterus:* Note shape, masses	Smooth, uniform, no masses	Masses, irregular shape
• *Rectal wall:* Note masses, tenderness, tone (obtain stool specimen from gloved hand)	Smooth, nontender, firm muscle tone	Nodules, masses, lesions Tender Absent tone

▮ Physical Assessment: External and Internal Structures

Pediatric Adaptations

INFANT

Steps	Normal and/or Common Findings	Significant Deviations
Inspection		
• *Discharge:* Note presence	Absent or slight white discharge or blood in first week	
• *Labia:* Note size, position	Edematous, slightly opened	Ambiguous genitalia
• *Vaginal opening:* Note presence	Patent	Absence of vaginal opening
• *Anus*	Meconium passed in first 24 hours	No meconium in first 24 hours

Physical Assessment: External and Internal Structures

Pediatric Adaptations

CHILD

Steps	Normal and/or Common Findings	Significant Deviations
Inspection Note: complete gynecologic examinations, including Pap smear, should begin when individual becomes sexually active or at age 18–20		
• Hair growth	No hair; preadolescent Slight fine hair on labia majora; hair darker, thicker but finer texture and amount less than adult	Pubic hair before 9 years old
• *Genital region:* Note signs of sexual abuse	No signs of abuse Hymenal tag	Scarring, lesions, red or darkened pigment, poor sphincter tone, vaginal odor (and other signs of infection), bleeding, pain, presence of STDs

Physical Assessment: External and Internal Structures

Geriatric Adaptations

Steps	Normal and/or Common Findings	Significant Deviations
Inspection • External genitalia	Atrophied; diminished fat pads; sparse, white hair	Masses, lesions, nodules, inflammation, gross asymmetry, erythema

(Continued on following page)

(Continued)

Steps	Normal and/or Common Findings	Significant Deviations
Inspection (Continued)		
• Mucosa	Pale, thin, friable	Tears, lesions, erythematous
• Secretions, discharges	Scanty to absent	Colored, malodorous, or abundant discharges, **urinary incontinence**
• Uterus, ovaries	Nontender, atrophied, smaller; ovaries not palpable	Pain, asymmetry, enlarged, rectocele, cystocele, uterine prolapse

▧ Physical Assessment: External Structures

Cultural Adaptations

Steps	Normal and/or Common Findings	Significant Deviations
Inspection		
• Labia majora	Darker pigmentation	

▧ Diagnostic Tests

May need to refer for:

- Pap smear
- <u>Other smears and cultures:</u> Gonococcal culture, DNA probe for gonorrhea and *Chlamydia*, wet and dry mounts for other microbes
- Guaiac test of stool
- <u>Urodynamic testing:</u> Comprehensive workup for urinary and/or fecal incontinence
- Sexual dysfunction workup

Possible Nursing Diagnoses

- Pain, acute or chronic
- Rape-trauma syndrome
- Self-care deficit, bathing/hygiene
- Sexual dysfunction
- Sexuality pattern, altered

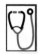

Clinical Alert

- Signs of sexual assault
- Masses
- Unusual pain
- Postmenopausal bleeding
- Infection signs and symptoms
- Pregnancy signs
- Urinary frequency, urgency, dysuria, or new urinary incontinence

Sample Documentation

Adult

- External genitalia nontender, not inflamed; normal hair distribution. Vaginal mucosa pink, moist, smooth. Cervix nulliparous, pink, without ulcers or nodules, nontender with movement. Pap smear obtained. Uterus palpable, nonenlarged, without masses or tenderness. Ovaries small and nontender. Rectum without hemorrhoids, masses, tenderness. Rectal wall smooth, firm, non-tender. Sphincter tone strong.

Child

- Tanner stage I. Labia pink and moist, no discharge.

▧ Patient Education and Home Health Notes

- Teach proper hygiene and prevention of cystitis and vaginitis:
  - Cleanse front to back.
  - Wear loose clothing, as few layers as possible.
  - Wear cotton underpants; avoid pantyhose when possible.
  - Urinate after intercourse.
  - Avoid tub baths, bubble bath, strongly perfumed soaps and powders.
  - Never use vaginal deodorants, deodorized tampons, or pads.
  - Avoid vaginal douches.
  - Drink more fluids (>8 glasses per day) if a history of cystitis.
- Pap smear schedule: After two normal smears, repeat every 2 to 3 years until age 40 if not at high risk (multiple partners, early onset of sexual activity, family history of cancer). Every year after age 40.
- Teach about contraception.
- Teach prevention of STDs: Limit activity to one mutually monogamous, uninfected partner; use condom with every exposure; emphasize risk of multiple partners (both STDs and cervical cancer), and risk of partners who use injected drugs
- Health-care workers at risk for exposure to blood-borne pathogens, who receive blood transfusions, engage in unprotected sexual activity, have multiple sexual partners, or use intravenous drugs should have hepatitis B series. Institutionalized mentally ill persons and those on hemodialysis should also be immunized.
- Explain risks of STDs.
- Teach prevention of HIV:
  - People become infected with HIV by having, oral, anal or vaginal sex with someone who has HIV

(Continued on following page)

- If sexually active, have oral, anal, or vaginal intercourse only with one mutually monogamous partner who does not use injection drugs and who is not infected with HIV. Emphasize risks of having multiple sex partners.
- Learn to correctly use latex barrier protection, like condoms, each and every time having oral, anal, or vaginal intercourse.
- Do not have sex with multiple partners, with persons who have multiple partners, with persons who use injected drugs, or with persons who have or are at risk for having HIV infection.
- Do not use drugs that can affect judgment, resulting in unsafe sex.
- Do not share needles. This includes needles used for injecting drugs, vitamins, or steroids and needles used for tattooing and body piercing. Do not share the equipment or "works" for preparing injected drugs.
- Do not share razors or toothbrushes.
- Those who have had unprotected sex or shared needles with anyone should have an HIV test.

Pediatric

- Teach proper hygiene as outlined above.
- Teach about contraception and STD prevention as indicated by age and sexual activity.
- Teach parents and child techniques in self-protection; for example, always tell parent or another adult if touched, threatened, or hurt. Assertively refuse to be touched, looked at, or show intimate parts. Tell child that sexual assault is the fault of the adult, not the child.

- Teach about normal changes associated with aging, for example, need for water-soluble lubricant for intercourse.
- Review all precautions for preventing STDs and HIV.
- Explain that sexual activity is normal into a person's 80s or 90s and beyond if there are no major health problems that interfere.
- Explain that persons with chronic illnesses may need to find alternative positions for sexual intercourse (e.g., side-lying position for patient with arthritis) and/or alternative methods for sexual enjoyment (e.g., kissing, caressing, manual stimulation).
- Inform patient that fecal and urinary incontinence are treatable conditions and that it is crucial for patient to seek help from a health-care provider early. If the health-care provider does not respond to requests for investigation and assistance with incontinence problems, tell patient to seek help from a specialist, such as a urologist, a geriatrician, or an advanced practice nurse who specializes in such problems.
- Explain that pelvic examinations by health-care professionals should be performed annually and Pap smears performed as indicated.
- Urinary Incontinence (Table 20–1) transient causes:
  - Delirium, acute confusion
  - UTI
  - Atrophic vaginitis or urethritis
  - Severe depression
  - Excessive urine production, diuresis
  - Limited mobility
  - Constipation
  - <u>Medications:</u> Sedative hypnotics, diuretics, anticholinergics, psychotropics (Table 20–2)

Table 20-1

Types of Chronic Urinary Incontinence (UI)

—Stress UI	a. Leakage with cough, sneeze, physical activity b. UI in small amounts (drops, spurts)	c. No nocturia or UI at night d. UI without sensation of urine loss
—Urge UI	a. Strong, uncontrolled urge prior to UI b. Moderate/large volume of urine loss (gush)	c. Frequency of urination d. Nocturia >2 e. Enuresis
—Overflow UI	a. Difficulty starting urine stream b. Weak or intermittent stream (dribbles) with changes in position	c. Postvoid dribbling d. Feeling of fullness after voiding e. Voiding in small amount often or dribbling
—Functional UI	a. Mobility or manual dexterity impairments b. Sedative, hypnotic, central nervous system (CNS) depressant, diuretic, anticholinergic, alpha adrenergic antagonist	c. Depression, delirium, dementia d. Pain

Source: Adapted from Dash, ME, Foster, EB, Smith, DM, and Phillips, SL: Urinary Incontinence: The Social Health Maintenance Organization's Approach (CE). Geriatric Nursing, 25(2): 85, 2004. used with permission.

Table 20-2

Diagnosis and Treatment Interventions for Urinary Incontinence

Definition	**One or more urinary accidents in past month or complaints about the problem**

Diagnosis	1. Evaluate presence of:
	  a. Diabetes
	  b. Congestive heart failure (CHF)
	  c. Neurological lesions
	  d. Postgenitourinary (GU) surgery
	2. History (onset, pattern, fluid intake)
	3. Physical exam including:
	  a. Pelvic (female)
	  b. Prostate (male)
	  c. Urinalysis to rule out hematuria, infection
	  d. Postvoid residual

Treatment	4. Treat acute/episodic causes:
	  a. **D**elirium
	  b. **I**nfection
	  c. **A**trophic vaginitis
	  d. **P**harmaceuticals
	    i. Retention overflow
	      1. Antidepressants
	      2. Antipsychotics
	      3. Antidiarrhea drugs
	      4. Antiparkinsonian drugs
	      5. Decongestants
	      6. Calcium channel blockers
	      7. Alpha agonists (men)
	    ii. Urge incontinence
	      1. Alpha blockers
	      2. Diuretics
	      3. Parasympathomimetics
	  e. **P**sychological
	  f. **E**ndocrine
	  g. **R**estricted mobility
	  h. **S**tool impaction
	5. Treat chronic causes according to type:
	  a. Storage disorders—bladder size normal
	    i. Urge incontinence (detrusor overactivity): frequent voids, dry in between, variable amounts of leakage; treat with behavioral techniques, anticholinergics

(Continued on following page)

        ii. Stress incontinence: small leakage with cough, sneeze, etc.; treat with behavioral techniques, alpha agonists, estrogens, surgery, periurethral injection, pessary

        iii. Mixed (stress and urge): both symptoms/signs; treat with behavioral techniques, estrogens and imipramine, pessary

     b. Emptying disorders: distended bladder causes overflow incontinence; slow stream; frequent, small leakage; strain; hesitancy

        i. Detrusor underactivity: treat by maximizing cholinergic tone, avoid alpha stimulation

        ii. Outlet obstruction: treat with alpha blockade, 5-alpha reductase inhibitors, TURP, urethral dilation

Stress Incontinence Medications	Estrogen: Cream 1 g/d vaginally, 5x/wk
	Plus
	Alpha agonist (phenylpropanolamine 60 mg bid)
	OR
	Pseudoephedrine 30-60 mg tid
	OR
	Imipramine 10-25 mg tid
Behavioral Techniques	Scheduled voiding
	Habit training
	Pelvic strengthening (Kegel)
	Exercises
	Bladder drill (expand time between voids)
	Adequate/appropriate fluid intake
Urge Incontinence Medications	Oxybutynin 2.5 mg qd - 5 mg tid
	OR
	Imipramine 10-25 mg tid
	OR
	Ditropan XL 5-10 mg/day
Monitoring	Depends on treatment plan and patient response

*Source: Adapted from Dash, ME, Foster, EB, Smith, DM, and Phillips, SL:
Urinary Incontinence: The Social Health Maintenance Organization's Approach (CE).
Geriatric Nursing, 25(2): 83–84, 2004. used with permission.*

Associated Community Agencies

- Help for Incontinent People: Patient advocacy and education
- National Kidney Foundation: Local screening programs, education, and counseling
- National Kidney and Urologic Diseases Information Clearinghouse: Education

CHAPTER **21**

Pregnancy

History

Adult

Antepartum
- Age
- Last menstrual period (LMP)
- Menstrual history (See Female Genitourinary System and Rectum, p. 272.)
- Contraceptive history (See Female Genitourinary System and Rectum, p. 272.)
- Obstetric history: Gravidity, parity, number of preterm births, number of term births, number of living children. For each previous birth: Gestation, birth weight, length of labor, newborn problems, and problems during pregnancy or labor
- Number of abortions, spontaneous or induced, and gestation of each
- Health since LMP: If illnesses, nature and treatment
- Accident and/or trauma history since pregnancy or with previous pregnancies. If significant, explore possibility of battering.
- Use of tobacco, alcohol, any drugs since LMP: Note type, amount, frequency.
- Cat in home (concern about toxoplasmosis when changing kitty litter). *(Continued on following page)*

- Known genetic or chromosomal abnormalities of either parent or family
- Months attempted conception
- Weight at LMP
- Dietary pattern
- Date of quickening
- Problems with this pregnancy
- Daily routine
- Knowledge of pregnancy and normal changes
- Relationships with father of baby and other family; degree of perceived support
- Assess feelings toward pregnancy, planned or unplanned, current level of acceptance

Intrapartum

- Screening assessment and interview initially performed to determine imminent birth (obstetric triage data)
- Obstetric triage data include:
  - <u>Obstetric history:</u> Gravidity/parity (previous methods of delivery): LMP-estimated date of delivery (EDD) by dates or sonography
  - <u>Primary reason for coming to hospital seeking care:</u> Onset of labor. Induction of labor, cesarean section, preterm labor, vaginal bleeding, rupture of membranes
  - <u>Contractions:</u> Frequency, duration, intensity, onset time, and date
  - <u>Membranes:</u> Intact, ruptured (date, time, amount, color, odor)
  - <u>Vaginal bleeding:</u> Mixed with mucus (bloody show), color, amount, onset
  - <u>Cervical exam:</u> Station, effacement, dilation, presentation
  - Fetal heart assessment and maternal vital signs
  - Admission physical assessment
- <u>Allergies:</u> Medications, other (remember latex sensitivity)
- Additional interview data
  - Recent illness ≤14 days before admission
  - Recent exposure to communicable disease
  - <u>Last oral intake:</u> Food/solids
  - Medications

(Continued on following page)

- • <u>Plans for birth and hospital stay:</u> Support person in labor and delivery; anesthesia: type; adoption; feeding preference; tubal ligation; circumcision
- Psychosocial data
  - Communication deficit
  - Partner/others involved
  - <u>Basic needs met:</u> Housing, clothing, food, transportation
  - Free from physical/emotional abuse
  - <u>Life stress:</u> Living environment, working, serious illness
  - <u>Self-care needs:</u> Able to meet, deficits
  - <u>Emotional status:</u> Happy, ambivalent, anxious, depressed, angry
- Significant prenatal data (the following should be available at admission):
  - Date of first prenatal visit
  - Previous medical history: significant family medical history
  - Prenatal classes/prepared childbirth
  - Lab findings on prenatal record
  - Blood type and Rh; rubella titer; serology; HIV status; hepatitis B surface antigen; GBS status
  - Maternal problems identified
  - Fetal problems identified

Postpartum

- Delivery date, length of labor, route of delivery, complications, status of infant
- Breast or bottle feeding
- Adequacy or difficulty in self-care (specify)
- <u>Adequacy or difficulty in newborn care:</u> Feeding, bathing, dressing, comforting
- Ability of support person to assist in care of mother and infant
- Contraception planned

- Perception of pregnancy as natural and healthy or as illness, source of pride or shame

(Continued on following page)

- Meaning and value of children, gender preference
- Roles of mother and father in family
- Common beliefs and practices related to childbearing, for example, raising hands above head may cause nuchal cord, attending funerals may expose fetus to evil spirits, open windows at night expose fetus to "bad air," pregnant woman attending wedding may bring bad luck to couple, temperature of foods may be significant in postpartum period
- Use of alternative health-care resources such as herbalist, spiritualist, Mexican curandero
- Family and individual roles that may influence decision making, teaching, delivery of care, expression of concerns; for example, mother may defer to father in decision making, father may be reluctant to express fear and anxiety, use of female caregiver may be necessary, significant inclusion of extended family in childbirth

Equipment

- Stethoscope
- Sphygmomanometer
- Centimeter tape
- Fetoscope (fetal Doppler if available)
- Speculum
- Glove
- Urinalysis for glucose, protein

Patient Preparation

- Have patient in sitting and lying positions.
- Have patient empty bladder and obtain clean urine specimen.
- Use supine position as little as possible.

Physical Assessment: Pregnancy

On admission, order of physical assessment is based upon factors surrounding labor, quick assessment of fetal status, fetal position and presentation, and vaginal exam to rule out imminent birth.

Steps	Normal and/or Common Findings	Significant Deviations
Antepartum Assessment		
Inspection		
• *Face and head:* Note color, pigmentation, edema	Chloasma, no edema, nasal stuffiness	Edema, especially periorbital and around bridge of nose
• *Breasts:* Note size, vascularity, color	Increased size, visible vessels symmetrical darkened areolar areas	Pain, redness, warmth
• *Abdomen:* Note size, shape, color striae, umbilical flattening	Size (Fig. 21–1); ovoid shape, striae, linea nigra may be present; umbilicus flattens after 30 weeks	Size not appropriate to gestational age
• *Cervix:* Note color, shape of os, discharge	Dark pink to blue (at 8–12 weeks); softened; os closed in nulliparas; slitlike opening in multiparas; no bleeding; increased white creamy discharge	Frank bleeding not associated with examination or intercourse
• Musculoskeletal	Increased lumbar curve and waddling gait in last trimester; mild dependent edema with prolonged standing	Marked dependent edema
Palpation		
• *Abdomen:* Note size, pain	Fundal height palpable after 12–13 weeks (see Fig. 21–1)	Fundal height not appropriate to gestational age; painful to palpate
• *Neurologic:* Note reflex irritability	Reflexes +2. No clonus	Reflexes +3 or +4; clonus of ankle

(Continued on page 294)

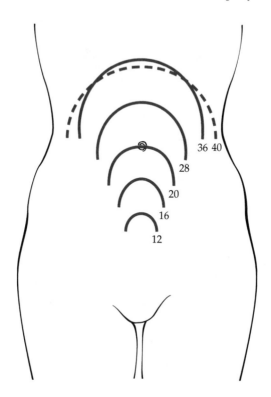

Figure 21-1 Fundal heights and gestation.

(Continued)

Steps	Normal and/or Common Findings	Significant Deviations
Antepartum Assessment		
Auscultation		
• *Heart:* Note rate, other sounds	Rate may increase 10–15 beats per minute; may have short systolic murmurs	Tachycardia; marked murmurs, palpitations
• *Blood pressure*	First and third trimesters at prepregnant level; falls in second trimester	>140/90 or systolic increase of 30 mm Hg; diastolic increase of 15 mm Hg (If elevated, turn to left side; test urine for protein.)
• *Fetal heart:* Note rate, rhythm, location (on mother's abdomen as RUQ, RLQ, LUQ, LLQ)	>160 at 12 weeks decreasing to 110–160 in late pregnancy; increases 15 beats per minute with activity; regular or slightly irregular rhythm	Not audible after 12 weeks with Doppler; not audible after 18–20 weeks with fetoscope Rate <110–120 in last trimester; no increase in rate with fetal movement; nonreassuring pattern or irregularity
Initial Intrapartum Assessment		
Inspection		
• *General appearance:* Look for signs of distress	Appearance and behavior varies depending on stage and phase of labor	Birth practices in different cultures; vary with cultural groups and different religions
• *Face and head:* Note color, edema	No edema, nasal stuffiness	*Edema:* especially periorbital and around bridge of nose
• *Breasts:* Note size, vascularity, color	Increased size, visible vessels symmetrical, darkened areolar areas	*Pain, redness,* warmth
• *Abdomen:* Note size, shape, color, striae, umbilicus flattening	*Size:* ovoid shape, striae, linea nigra may be present; umbilicus flattens after 30 weeks	*Size not appropriate to gestational age*

(Continued on following page)

Steps	Normal and/or Common Findings	Significant Deviations
Palpation		
• *Abdomen:* Note size, fetal positioning/presentation, pain, uterine activity	Fundal height palpation initially done for size estimation, Leopold's maneuvers; evaluation of labor contractions	Fundal height not appropriate to gestational age; fetal presentation other than vertex; uterine tone rigid without relaxing; extremely painful to palpate
• *Neurologic:* Note reflex irritability	Reflexes +2; no clonus	*Reflexes* +3 or +4; clonus of ankle
• *Vaginal examination:* Cervical dilation and effacement; fetal station and presentation; inspection of vaginal secretions	Vaginal examination dependent on stage and phase of labor	Bloody show in absence of pain; abnormal fetal presentation; presence of umbilical cord with presenting part; amniotic fluid with foul odor or meconium stained
Auscultation		
• *Heart:* Note rate, rhythm, presence of murmur	Rate may increase 10–15 beats per minute above non-pregnant rate; may have short systolic murmur	Tachycardia; marked murmurs
• *Blood pressure:* See vital signs	Will increase during contractions—check without contraction for accuracy	Palpitations Blood pressure readings of ≥30 mm Hg increase over systolic baseline, ≥15 mm Hg increase over diastolic baseline or reading of 140/90 mm Hg × 2–6 hours apart
• *Lungs:* Note breath sounds, adventitious sounds	Lung fields clear	Any adventitious breath sounds; hyperventilation

(Continued on following page)

(Continued)

Steps	Normal and/or Common Findings	Significant Deviations
Initial Intrapartum Assessment		
Auscultation (Continued)		
• *Fetal heart rate (FHR):* Note rate, rhythm, location (on mother's abdomen as RUQ, RLQ, LUQ, LLQ), FHR response to contractions	*Reassuring FHR patterns:* Baseline 110–160 beats per minute; average variability 6–25 beats per minute; no nonreassuring periodic changes; acceleration of FHR with fetal movement reassuring	Rate <110 beats per minute; variability consistently <6 beats per minute; no increase in rate with fetal activity *Nonreassuring periodic changes:* Late decelerations: FHR decelerations that begin after peak of contraction, lasting after contraction is over; prolonged decelerations: >2 minutes and <10 minutes; bradycardia: deceleration >10 minutes; tachycardia: >160 Severe variable decelerations, FHR <60 beats per minute, ≥60 seconds or variable decelerations with increasing baseline and decreasing variability associated with neonatal depression
Vital signs		
• Initial assessment should be used as baseline, as labor progresses	Temperature monitored every 4 hours; if membranes ruptured, every 2 hours	Temperature >100 Possible infection or fluid deficit
	Pulse and respiration monitored every 30–60 minutes in latent phase (early labor); every 15–30 minutes in transition phase	Tachycardia, tachypnea
	Blood pressure (should be at prepregnant level by 28 weeks) monitored same as pulse and respiration (if epidural anesthetic, every 15 minutes)	>140/90 or systolic increase of 30 mm Hg; diastolic increase of 15 mm Hg (if elevated, turn to left side, test urine for protein)

Physical Assessment: Pregnancy

	Intrapartum: Expected Maternal Progress During Labor					
	Stage 1*†			Stage 2‡	Stage 3	Stage 4
• Dilatation	0–3 cm (latent)	4–7 cm (active)	8–10 cm (transition)	Pushing—delivery of baby	Placental expulsion	2 hours postpartum
• Duration	About 6–8 hours	About 3–6 hours	About 20–40 minutes	Nullipara 25–75 minutes; average 57 minutes Multipara 13–17 minutes; average 14	5–30 minutes	
• Contractions Strength	Mild to moderate	Moderate to strong	Strong to very strong	Strong to very strong	Very strong	Afterbirth pains Mild
Rhythm Frequency	Irregular 5–30 minutes apart	More regular 3–5 minutes apart	Regular 2–3 minutes apart	Regular 2–3 minutes apart	Regular 1 1/2-3 minutes apart	Irregular Uterus must remain firm to decrease postpartum bleeding
• Duration	30–45 seconds	40–70 seconds	45–90 seconds	90 seconds	60–90 seconds	
• Station: descent of presenting part	Nullip: 0 Multip: 0–2 cm	Varies +1 cm to +2 cm	Varies +2 cm to +3 cm	0 to +2 → +4 at birth		

(Continued on following page)

	Stage 1*†		Stage 2‡	Stage 3	Stage 4
Color	Brown discharge, mucus plug or pale pink mucus	Pink to bloody mucus	Bloody mucus	Significant increase in dark red bloody show → fetal head at introitus; bloody show at birth	Gushing of dark blood; cord lengthens	Lochia-rubra-like heavy menses with clots
Amount	Scant	Scant to moderate	Copious			
• Behavior and appearance	Excited—Self-control, thinking of baby, pain fairly well controlled; follows directions	More serious, more apprehensive; wants encouragement; focused inwardly; some difficulty following directions	Pain—Severe, frustration, fear of loss of control; irritable; nausea and vomiting; feels need to defecate	Relief, fatigue—sleepy; "worst is over"; feels in control → extreme pain; decreased ability to listen; focused on giving birth; extreme excitement after delivery of head	Relief—Crying, laughing, concern for baby	Many factors affect mother: low energy level, physical comfort, health of newborn; transitioning

Intrapartum: Expected Maternal Progress During Labor (Continued)

*In nulliparous women, effacement usually complete before dilatation begins; in multiparous women effacement and dilatation occur simultaneously. Average total duration of stage 1 nullipara 10–16 hours; multipara 6–10 hours.
†Duration of first and second stage of labor influenced by parity, maternal position and activity. Nullipara's labor > multipara's labor.
‡Length of time during second stage lengthens with epidural anesthesia.

Physical Assessment: Pregnancy

Steps	Normal and/or Common Findings	Significant Deviations
Postpartum Assessment		
Inspection		
• *Breasts:* Note color, feeding ability	No redness; infant able to root, grasp areolar tissue in mouth, suck 5 minutes each side first days in at least two positions	Redness Infant unable to suck 5 minutes each side
• *Abdomen:* Note uterine, bladder positions	Not visible or midline, below umbilicus	Easily visible above umbilicus or deviated laterally
• *Perineum:* Note color, integrity, swelling, drainage	Slight redness, mild edema, lochia appropriate to time (rubra to serosa) If episiotomy, no signs of infection of incision If hemorrhoids, may be swollen	Bright red or unilateral redness; continued lochia rubra beyond first days; strong odor Bright red bleeding; signs of infection of episiotomy
Palpation		
• *Breast* (wash hands before touching): Note warmth, hard areas, tenderness or pain	Mild uniform warmth; no masses; some tenderness, especially nipples	Hot areas, hardened areas, painful to touch
• *Abdomen:* Note fundal height, firmness; bladder tenderness	*Day 1:* At umbilicus, firm *Day 2:* Umbilicus +1 to 2 cm *Day 3:* At umbilicus *Day 4:* Steady decrease Bladder not palpable	Fundus boggy, elevated, deviated laterally; bladder palpable with suprapubic tenderness
• *Legs:* Gently palpate calves for heat, tenderness; dorsiflex ankle, and ask patient if pain felt in calf	No heat No pain (negative Homans' sign)	Heat, pain on dorsiflexion (positive Homans' sign)
• *Skin:* Note temperature, moisture	Warm (oral temperature <100.4°F); increased perspiration	Temperature >100.4°F

📖 Diagnostic Tests

- Initial prenatal tests include: CBC, urinalysis, serology, HIV, rubella screen, blood type, Rh and antibody screen, hepatitis B surface antigen, DNA probe for chlamydia and gonorrhea, Pap smear. Possibly culture for group B streptococcus.
- Diabetic screen in 2nd trimester
- Ultrasonography
- Pelvimetry
- Quad-marker blood test offered as screen for certain fetal problems (e.g., neural tube defects) in second trimester

📖 Possible Nursing Diagnoses

- Sleep pattern disturbance
- Breastfeeding, effective, ineffective, interrupted
- Knowledge deficit (learning need) (specify)
- Fatigue
- Growth and development, altered
- Body image disturbance
- Nutrition: altered, more or less than body requirements
- Family processes, altered

Clinical Alert

- Elevated blood pressure, facial edema, proteinuria, glucosuria, headache
- Nonreassuring fetal heart pattern
- Uterine growth disproportionate to gestational age
- Mother's report of decreased fetal movement
- Bleeding not associated with examination or intercourse
- Abdominal pain

🔖 Sample Documentation

Age 33; G-2, T-1, P-0, A-0, L-1. Approximately 22 weeks gestation (LMP 5/26; EDD 2/28). Fundus at umbilicus 20 cm, FHR 170 LLQ. Urine neg/neg; weight 158; BP 100/70. Bimanual; Cervix closed, soft, thick. Speculum: Cervix closed, without lesions or drainage.

🔖 Patient and Family Education and Home Health Notes

- Teach normal changes of pregnancy, and maternal and fetal development.
- Review dietary needs every month. Assess with recall if weight gain too much or too little.
- Encourage moderate exercise (e.g., walking, swimming) and rest.
- Explain that normal weight gain is from 24 to 32 pounds. During first 28 weeks, patient should gain 1/2 to 3/4 pound per week; then she should gain from 1 to 1 1/2 pounds per week.
- Teach danger signs in pregnancy.
- Teach warning signs of labor.
- Teach infant care and infant normal growth and development.
- Discuss breast-feeding and provide information and support. Provide information about bottle feeding if desired.
- Discuss return to sexual activity.
- Teach patient when to see health-care provider postpartum (baby is normally seen at 2 weeks, mother at 6 weeks).
- Assess and provide information about sibling preparation.
- Assess adequacy of infant care supplies:
  - Crib or bassinet
  - Car seat
  - Infant clothing, diapers, feeding materials
- Assess availability of support person for labor and postpartum.

■ Associated Community Agencies

- Prenatal classes
- Family resource centers
- Licensed breastfeeding specialists
- Local support agencies for new parents and breastfeeding mothers
- Supplemental Nutrition Program for Women, Infants, and Children (WIC)
- Food stamps
- Temporary Aid to Needy Families (TANF)
- La Leche League
- Parenting classes
- Breastfeeding classes

APPENDIX A

NANDA-APPROVED NURSING DIAGNOSES

Nursing Diagnoses through the 14th NANDA Conference in Alphabetical Order

Activity intolerance (specify level)
Activity intolerance, risk for
Adaptive capacity: Intracranial, decreased
Adjustment, impaired
Airway clearance, ineffective
Anxiety
Anxiety, death
Aspiration, risk for
Body image disturbance
Body temperature, risk for altered
Bowel incontinence
Breastfeeding, effective
Breastfeeding, ineffective
Breastfeeding, interrupted
Breathing pattern, ineffective
Cardiac output, decreased
Caregiver role strain
Caregiver role strain, risk for
Communication, impaired verbal
Community coping, ineffective
Community coping, potential for enhanced
Confusion, acute
Confusion, chronic
Constipation
Constipation, perceived
Risk of constipation
Coping, defensive
Coping, individual, ineffective

Source: NANDA International (2002). NANDA Nursing Diagnoses: Definitions and Classification 2003–2004. Philadelphia: NANDA.

Decisional conflict (specify)
Denial, ineffective
Dentition, altered
Development, risk for altered
Diarrhea
Disorganized infant behavior
Disorganized infant behavior, risk for
Disuse syndrome, risk for
Diversional activity deficit
Dysreflexia
Dysreflexia, risk for autonomic
Energy field disturbance
Enhanced organized infant behavior, potential for
Environmental interpretation syndrome, impaired
Failure to thrive, adult
Falls, risk for
Family coping, ineffective: Compromised
Family coping, ineffective: Disabling
Family coping: Potential for growth
Family processes, altered
Family process, altered: Alcoholism (substance abuse)
Fatigue
Fear
Fluid volume deficit, hyper/hypotonic
Fluid volume deficit, isotonic
Fluid volume deficit, risk for
Fluid volume excess
Fluid volume imbalance, risk for
Gas exchange, impaired
Grieving, anticipatory
Grieving, dysfunctional
Growth and development, altered
Growth, risk for altered
Health maintenance, altered
Health-seeking behaviors (specify)
Home maintenance management, impaired
Hopelessness
Hyperthermia
Hypothermia
Incontinence, functional urinary
Incontinence, reflex urinary
Incontinence, stress

Incontinence, total
Incontinence, urge
Incontinence, risk for urinary urge
Infant feeding pattern, ineffective
Infection, risk for
Injury, risk for
Knowledge deficit: Learning need (specify)
Latex allergy response
Latex allergy response, risk for
Loneliness, risk for
Memory, impaired
Mobility, impaired bed
Mobility, impaired physical
Mobility, impaired wheelchair
Nausea
Noncompliance/compliance, altered (specify)
Nutrition: Altered, less than body requirements
Nutrition: Altered, more than body requirements
Nutrition: Altered, risk for more than body requirements
Oral mucous membrane, altered
Pain, acute
Pain, chronic
Parent/infant/child attachment, altered, risk for
Parent-infant attachment, risk for insecure
Parental role conflict
Parenting, altered
Parenting, risk for altered
Perioperative positioning injury, risk for
Peripheral neurovascular, risk for dysfunction
Personal identity disturbance
Poisoning, risk for
Post-trauma syndrome
Post-trauma syndrome, risk for
Powerlessness (specify level)
Powerlessness, risk for
Protection, altered
Rape-trauma syndrome
Rape-trauma syndrome: Compound reaction
Rape-trauma syndrome: Silent reaction
Recovery, delayed surgical
Relocation stress syndrome
Relocation stress syndrome, risk for

Role performance, altered
Self-care deficit, feeding
Self-care deficit, bathing/hygiene
Self-care deficit, dressing/grooming
Self-care deficit, toilet
Self-esteem, chronic, low
Self-esteem disturbance
Self-esteem, situational, low
Self-esteem, situational low, risk for
Self-mutilation
Self-mutilation, risk for
Sensory/perceptual alterations (specify): Visual, auditory, kinesthetic, gustatory, tactile, olfactory
Sexual dysfunction
Sexuality pattern, altered
Skin integrity, impaired
Skin integrity, impaired, risk for
Sleep deprivation
Sleep pattern disturbance
Social interaction, impaired
Social isolation
Sorrow, chronic
Spiritual distress (distress of the human spirit)
Spiritual distress, risk for
Spiritual well-being, enhanced, potential for
Spontaneous ventilation, inability to sustain
Suffocation, risk for
Suicide, risk for
Swallowing, impaired
Therapeutic regimen (community), ineffective management of
Therapeutic regimen (families), ineffective management of
Therapeutic regimen (individual), effective management of
Therapeutic regimen (individual), ineffective management of
Thermoregulation, ineffective
Thought processes, altered
Tissue integrity, impaired
Tissue perfusion, altered (specify type): Renal, cerebral, cardiopulmonary, gastrointestinal, peripheral
Transfer ability, impaired
Trauma, risk for
Unilateral neglect
Urinary elimination, altered patterns of

Urinary retention (acute/chronic)
Ventilatory weaning response, dysfunctional (DVWR)
Violence, actual/risk for, directed at others
Violence, actual/risk for, self-directed
Walking, impaired
Wandering (specify sporadic or continual)

APPENDIX B

Age Categories and Labels and Words Used for Older People

Age Categories

Young-old	65–74
Middle-old	75–84
Old-old	85–94
Elite-old	95 and older

Functional status is more important than chronologic age. Categories provided by the National Institute on Aging, August 30, 1994.

Labels and Words

Words and terms that should not be used when talking with or about or writing about the disabled or older people. Many of the terms are disrespectful and demeaning. Others have *unclear meanings* open to various interpretations.

DO NOT USE	SUBSTITUTE
• Adult day care (similar to child care)	Adult day services (may include needed health care)
• Adult diaper (implies being a baby)	Pants, pads, briefs, trade name (product)
• Afflicted	Affected by
• Aged	Older people
• Bedbound (not tied to the bed)	In bed much of the time
• Bed sore	Pressure ulcer (area)
• Bib	Clothes protector

(Continued on following page)

DO NOT USE	**SUBSTITUTE** *(Continued)*
• Cerebral palsied	People with cerebral palsy
• Childish, childlike, baby	None (never use)
• Convalescent home	Nursing facility
• Crazy, insane, psycho, maniac	People with mental illness/behavioral problems
• Crippled	People with disabilities
• Deaf and dumb, mute	Hearing and speech impaired
• Elderly (implies 50–110 all alike)	Older people
• First name or familial title (granny)	Only if family, friend, or by request
• Formula (relates to babies)	Nutritional supplement
• Frail, fragile (what does this mean?)	Describe specific problem
• Golden agers	None (never use)
• Greedy geezers (means odd character of any age)	None (never use)
• Handicapped or disabled	People with disabilities
• Homebound, shut-in (not tied to the house)	Rarely leaves home
• Honey, dearie, sweetie, grandpa, grandma	Mr., Ms., Dr.
• Incompetent (old legal term)	Incapacitated (determined by the courts based on the physician's assessment)
• Little old lady (man)— what does little mean?	Older woman (man)
• Oldsters	Older people
• Old timer's disease (implying Alzheimer's/bad joke)	None (never use)
• Poor	Low income
• Rest home	Nursing facility (home)
• Role reversal (dependent parent becomes child)	Role reversal does not occur (a mature adult-to-adult relationship)

(Continued on following page)

DO NOT USE	SUBSTITUTE
• Senile (implies confusion)	None (never use)
• Senior (many uses for this word)	Older adult
• Senior moment (implies forgetfulness/bad joke)	Never use (all ages forget at times)
• Sitter (used for babies)	Companion
• Suffers (from a disease)	Has a disease
• Symptoms/problems caused by age	Diagnose and treat
• Victim (of a disease)	None (never use)
• Wheelchair bound (not tied to the wheelchair)	Wheelchair user
• Young man (lady)—when obviously older	None (never use)

Source: Adapted from Hogstel, MO: Community Resources for Older Adults: A Guide for Case Managers. St Louis: Mosby. 1998, with permission.
Note: Some words have been contributed by REACH, a Resource Center on Independent Living in Fort Worth, Texas and the Texas Council for Developmental Disabilities, Austin, Texas.

Sample Health History Form

Date _____ Name _____

Room _____ Sex: M F

Address _____

Telephone number _____

Private home _____ Apartment _____

Retirement center _____ Nursing facility _____

Date of birth _____ Age _____

Date of admission _____ Date of surgery _____

Marital status: M W S D

If widowed, how long? _____

Retired _____ Occupation _____

Medicare number _____

Medicaid number _____

Insurance name _____

Number _____

Religious preference _____

Contact in emergency _____

Source: Adapted from Nursing History From 584, Harris School of
Nursing. Texas Christian University. Fort Worth. TX, 2004, with
permission.

Reason for seeking care (chief complaint) _____

_____

History of present illness/condition/surgery _____

_____

_____

_____

Patient's understanding of current condition _____

_____

Current diet _____

Medications currently prescribed _____

_____

Past health/medical history _____

_____

_____

_____

Allergies (food, medicines, environmental) _____

_____

_____

Medications and treatments at home _____

_____

Chemical use

Number of cigarettes per day _____

Other tobacco per day _____

Number of years smoked _____

Amount of coffee/tea/carbonated beverages per day _____

Amount of alcoholic drinks per day _____

Type _____

Use of other substances _____

_____

Rest and sleep patterns

Hours worked per day _____ Rest periods or naps (when, _____)

Hours of sleep per night _____

Medications used to aid sleep _____

Other measures to aid sleep _____

Sleep problems _____

_____

Mobility and exercise patterns

Type of activity/exercise _____

Amount (times per week, minutes per day) _____

Restrictions/mechanical aids/prostheses/wheelchair/walker/
bedrails _____

Ability to care for self _____

_____

Diet

	Breakfast	*Lunch*	*Dinner*	*Snacks*
24-hour recall of previous day				
Usual time of meals at home				

Ability to feed self_____ Dentures _____

Frequency of dental examinations/difficulties _____

Dietary restrictions/dislikes, difficulty_____

Fluid intake per day (type and amount)_____

Elimination routines, frequency, problems, aids

Bowel _____

_____

Urinary _____

_____

Communication

Ability to understand English _____

Language spoken _____

Hearing _____ Sight _____ Aids _____

Educational level _____

Ability to speak _____

Orientation: Person _____ Time _____

Place _____

Present emotional state _____

Activities

Hobbies _____

Part-time employment _____

Volunteer work _____

Other _____

Family history
Composition
   Number in household
   Roles
Primary support system
History of family health/illness
Other pertinent data

Environmental history

◼ Review of Systems

System	History	Not Asked
General overview		
Skin/hair/nails		
Head and Neck		
Eyes		
Ears		
Nose/sinus		
Mouth/throat		
Respiratory		

(Continued on following page)

(Continued)

System	History	Not Asked
Cardiovascular		
Gastrointestinal		
Breasts/axillae		
Genitourinary		
Musculoskeletal		
Neurologic		
Other pertinent data		

Sample Mental Status Assessment Flow Sheet

Key

✓ Intact
L Limited
D Difficult
φ Absent

Suggested Schedule

Each shift or daily (hospital)
Monthly (nursing facility, home health agency)

Assessment*	Each Shift or Daily *or*						Weekly *or*						Monthly					
	Date	Date	Date				Date		Date		Date		Date		Date		Date	
	Time	Time	Time				A.M.	P.M.	A.M.	P.M.	A.M.	P.M.	A.M.	P.M.	A.M.	P.M.	A.M.	P.M.
1. Oriented to person a. First name																		
b. Last name																		
2. Oriented to place a. City																		
b. State																		
c. Name of facility																		
d. Address of facility																		
3. Oriented to time a. Year																		
b. Month																		
c. Date of month																		
d. Day of week																		
e. A.M. or P.M.																		

Assessment*	Each Shift or Daily or						Weekly or						Monthly					
	Date	Date	Date				Date		Date		Date		Date		Date		Date	
	Time	Time	Time	A.M.	P.M.	A.M.	P.M.	A.M.	P.M.	A.M.	P.M.	A.M.	P.M.	A.M.	P.M.	A.M.	P.M.	
4. Memory a. Immediate (minutes): Name three objects and ask to repeat in several minutes.																		
b. Recent (days): Ask what the person did yesterday afternoon.																		
c. Remote (years): Ask about year of marriage or president during World War II.																		
d. Old (not recalled recently): Ask names of teachers from grade school.																		

(Continued on following page)

(Continued)

Assessment*	Each Shift or Daily *or*						Weekly *or*						Monthly					
	Date	Date	Date				Date		Date		Date		Date		Date		Date	
	Time	Time	Time				A.M.	P.M.	A.M.	P.M.	A.M.	P.M.	A.M.	P.M.	A.M.	P.M.	A.M.	P.M.
5. Intelligence																		
a. Vocabulary: Ask to name several objects such as a pencil.																		
b. Calculations: Ask to add or subtract two numbers.																		
c. Construction: Ask to draw the face of a clock.																		
6. Abstract thinking																		
a. Proverbs: Ask the meaning of a proverb such as "When it rains, it pours."																		

Assessment*	Each Shift or Daily			Weekly						Monthly			
	Date / Time	Date / Time	Date / Time	Date A.M.	P.M.	Date A.M.	P.M.	Date A.M.	P.M.	Date A.M.	P.M.	Date A.M.	P.M.
b. Analogies: Ask how an apple and an orange are alike.													
7. Mental status test score a. MMSE† b. Other													

or (between Each Shift or Daily and Weekly, and between Weekly and Monthly)

* Suggestions for assessment are only examples. Many other similar ones may be used.
† See Appendix E.
Source: Adapted from Hogstel, MO: Assessing mental status. J Geront Nurs 17(5):43, 1991, with permission.

The Folstein Mini-Mental State Examination (Test of Cognitive Function)

Maximum Score	*Score*	*Orientation*
5	( )	What is the (year)(season)(date)(day)(month)?
5	( )	Where are we: (state)(county)(town) (hospital)(floor)?
		Registration
3	( )	Name 3 objects: 1 second to say each. Then ask the patient all 3 after you have said them. Give 1 point for each correct answer. Then repeat them until he learns all 3. Count trials and record. Trials _____
		Attention and Calculation
5	( )	Serial 7's. 1 point for each correct. Stop after 5 answers. Alternatively spell "world" backwards.
		Recall
3	( )	Ask for 3 objects repeated above. Give 1 point for each correct.
		Language
2	( )	Name a pencil and watch.
1	( )	Repeat the following: "No ifs, ands, or buts."
3	( )	Follow a 3 stage command: "Take a paper in your right hand, fold it in half, and put it on the floor."

(Continued on following page)

(Continued)

Score	Score	Orientation
1	( )	Read and obey the following:
		CLOSE YOUR EYES
1	( )	Write a sentence.
<u>1</u>	( )	Copy design.
30		

ASSESS level of consciousness along a continuum (alert, drowsy, stupor, coma)

Source: Adapted from Folstein, MF, Folstein, SE, and McHugh. PR: Mini-mental state. Journal of Psychiatric Research, 12(1):196–197, 1975. Used with permission.

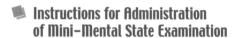

Instructions for Administration of Mini-Mental State Examination

Orientation

Ask for the date. Then ask specifically for parts omitted (e.g., "Can you also tell me what season it is?") One point for each correct.

Ask in turn "Can you tell me the name of this hospital?" (town, county, etc.). One point for each correct.

Registration

Ask the patient if you may test his memory. Then say the names of three unrelated objects, clearly and slowly, about one second for each. After you have said all three, ask him to repeat them. This first repetition determines his score (0–3), but keep saying them until he can repeat all three, up to six trials. If he does not eventually learn all three, recall cannot be meaningfully tested.

Attention and Calculation

Ask the patient to begin with 100 and count backwards by 7. Stop after 5 subtractions (93, 86, 79, 72, 65). Score the total number of correct answers.

If the patient cannot or will not perform this task, ask him to spell the word "world" backwards. The score is the number of letters in correct order (e.g., dlrow = 5, dlorw = 3).

Recall

Ask the patient if he can recall the three words you previously asked him to remember. Score 0–3.

Language

Naming: Show the patient a wrist watch and ask him what it is. Repeat for pencil. Score 0–2.

Repetition: Ask the patient to repeat the sentence after you. Allow only one trial. Score 0 or 1.

3-Stage command: Give the patient a piece of plain blank paper and repeat the command. Score 1 point for each part correctly executed (Folstein, et al., 1975, p. 197).

Scoring: A score of 20 or less has been found "only in patients with dementia, delirium, schizophrenia or affective disorders" (Folstein, et al., 1975, p. 196). The MMS is not timed and should only take about 5–10 minutes (Folstein, et al., 1975, p. 189).

References

Folstein, MF, Folstein, SE, and McHugh, PR: Mini-mental state. Journal of Psychiatric Research, 12(1):189–198, 1975.

Gallo, JJ, Reichel, W, and Andersen, LM: Handbook of Geriatric Assessment, Aspen, Gaithersburg, MD, 1995.

Note: Some changes in administration and scoring have occurred over the years based on research. Gallo, Reichel, and Andersen (1995, p. 33) used a "cutoff score of 24 … to indicate dementia." Scores may vary based on formal education completed and age.

Katz Index of Independence in Activities of Daily Living

The Index of Independence in Activities of Daily Living (ADLs) is based on an evaluation of the functional independence or dependence of patients in bathing, dressing, going to toilet, transferring, continence, and feeding. Specific definitions of functional independence and dependence appear after the index.

📰 Evaluation Form

Name _____ Date of evaluation _____

For each area of functioning listed below, check the one description that best applies. (The word *assistance* means supervision, direction of personal assistance.)

Bathing—either sponge bath, tub bath, or shower.

☐ Receives no assistance (gets into and out of tub by self if tub is usual means of bathing)	☐ Receives assistance in bathing only one part of the body (such as back or a leg)	☐ Receives assistance in bathing more than one part of the body (or not bathed)

Source: Adapted from Katz, S, Ford, AB, Moskowitz, RW, et al: Studies of illness in the aged: The Index of ADL. JAMA 185:914–919, 1963, with permission.

Dressing—gets clothes from closets and drawers including underclothes and outer garments and uses fasteners (including orthopedic braces if worn).

☐ Gets clothes and gets completely dressed without assistance	☐ Gets clothes and gets dressed without assistance except for assistance in tying shoes	☐ Receives assistance in getting clothes or in getting dressed, or stays partly or completely undressed

(Continued on following page)

(Continued)

Toileting—going to the "toilet room" for bowel and urine elimination; cleaning self after elimination, and arranging clothes.

☐ Goes to the "toilet room," cleans self, and arranges clothes without assistance (may use for support such object as cane, walker, or wheelchair and may manage night bedpan or commode, emptying same in morning)

☐ Receives assistance in going to "toilet room" or in cleansing self or in arranging clothes after elimination or in use of night bedpan or commode

☐ Does not go to room termed "toilet" for the elimination process

Transfers*

☐ Moves into and out of bed as well as into and out of chair without assistance (may be using object for support such as cane or walker)

☐ Moves into or out of bed or chair with assistance

☐ Does not get out of bed

---

* Ask the patient to show you the bathroom and medications in another room to assess ability to transfer, walk, and communicate.

Continence

☐ Controls urination and bowel movement completely by self

☐ Has occasional "accidents"

☐ Supervision to keep urine or bowel control; catheter used or is incontinent

Feeding

☐ Feeds self without assistance

☐ Feeds self except for getting assistance in cutting meat or buttering bread

☐ Receives assistance in feeding or is fed partly or completely by using tubes or intravenous fluids

---

Convert the above data into an overall ADL grade based on the following definitions. Note that the intermediate description may be dependent for some functions and independent for others.

A	Independent in feeding, continence, transferring, going to toilet, dressing, and bathing
B	Independent in all but one of these functions
C	Independent in all but bathing and one additional function
D	Independent in all but bathing, dressing, and one additional function
F	Independent in all but bathing, dressing, going to toilet, transferring, and one additional function
G	Dependent in all six functions
Other	Dependent in at least two functions but not classifiable as C, D, E, or F

Definitions

Independence means without supervision, direction, or active personal assistance, except as specifically noted below. This is based on actual status and not on ability. A patient who refuses to perform a function is considered as not performing the function, even though he or she is deemed able.

Bathing (Sponge, Shower, or Tub)

Independent. Assistance only in bathing a single part (as back or disabled extremity) or bathes self completely

Dependent. Assistance in bathing more than one part of body; assistance in getting into or out of tub or does not bathe self

Dressing

Independent. Gets clothes from closets and drawers; puts on clothes, outer garments, braces; manages fasteners (Act of trying shoes is excluded.)

Dependent. Does not dress self or remains partly undressed

Going to Toilet

Independent. Gets to toilet; gets on and off toilet; arranges clothes; cleans organs of excretion; may manage own bedpan used at night only and may or may not be using mechanical supports

Dependent. Uses bedpan or commode or receives assistance in getting to and using toilet

TRANSFER

Independent. Moves into and out of bed independently and moves into and out of chair independently; may or may not be using mechanical supports

Dependent. Assistance in moving into or out of bed and/or chair; does not perform one or more transfers

CONTINENCE

Independent. Urination and defecation entirely self-controlled

Dependent. Partial or total incontinence in urination or defecation; partial or total control by enemas, catheters, or regulated use of urinals and/or bedpans

FEEDING

Independent. Gets food from plate or its equivalent into mouth (Precutting of meat and preparation of food, such as buttering bread, are excluded from evaluation.)

Dependent. Assistance in act of feeding (see above); does not eat at all or receives parenteral feeding

Apgar Scoring System: A Rapid Assessment Technique to Determine Need for Resuscitation at 1 and 5 Minutes after Birth

	0	1	2
Heart rate	None	<100	>100
Respiration	None	Slow or irregular	Cries or makes good effort
Muscle tone	Flaccid	Mild flexion of extremities	Active movement
Reflex response (insert catheter in nostril after clearing oropharynx)	No response	Slow movement or grimaces	Cries, coughs, or sneezes
Color*	Blue, pale	Extremities blue, body pink	Completely pink

*Skin color or its absence may not be a reliable guide in nonwhites, although melanin is less apparent at birth than later.

Source: Adapted from Taber's Cyclopedic Medical Dictionary, ed. 19. FA Davis, Philadelphia, 2001, 147. with permission.

Scoring: Score each assessment area as 0, 1, or 2, based on the above criteria. Add the total score including all areas.

Interpretation:

0–3 = poor condition
4–6 = fair condition
7–10 = good to excellent condition

Recommended Childhood, Adolescent, and Adult Immunization Schedule

Recommended Childhood and Adolescent Immunization Schedule
United States · July–December 2004

Vaccine ▼ / Age ▶	Birth	1 mo	2 mo	4 mo	6 mo	12 mo	15 mo	18 mo	24 mo	4-6 y	11-12 y	13-18 y
Hepatitis B[1]	HepB #1	HepB #2 *only if mother HBsAg (-)*			HepB #3						HepB series	
Diphtheria, Tetanus, Pertussis[2]			DTaP	DTaP	DTaP		DTaP	DTaP		DTaP	Td	Td
Haemophilus influenzae Type b[3]			Hib	Hib	Hib	Hib						
Inactivated Poliovirus			IPV	IPV	IPV		IPV			IPV		
Measles, Mumps, Rubella[4]						MMR #1				MMR #2	MMR #2	
Varicella[5]						Varicella				Varicella	Varicella	
Pneumococcal[6]			PCV	PCV	PCV	PCV	PCV		PCV	PCV	PPV	
Influenza[7]					Influenza (Yearly)					Influenza (Yearly)		
Hepatitis A[8]											Hepatitis A Series	

Range of Recommended Ages · Catch-up Immunization · Preadolescent Assessment

– – – Vaccines below red line are for selected populations

This schedule indicates the recommended ages for routine administration of currently licensed childhood vaccines, as of April 1, 2004, for children through age 18 years. Any dose not given at the recommended age should be given at any subsequent visit when indicated and feasible. ▨ Indicates age groups that warrant special effort to administer those vaccines not previously given. Additional vaccines may be licensed and recommended during the year. Licensed combination vaccines may be used whenever any components of the combination are indicated and the vaccine's other components are not contraindicated. Providers should consult the manufacturers' package inserts for detailed recommendations. Clinically significant adverse events that follow immunization should be reported to the Vaccine Adverse Event Reporting System (VAERS). Guidance about how to obtain and complete a VAERS form can be found on the Internet: www.vaers.org or by calling 800-822-7967.

Recommended Adult Immunization Schedule — UNITED STATES • 2003-2004

Legend: For all persons in this group | Catch-up on childhood vaccinations | For persons with medical/exposure indications

VACCINE \ AGE	19-49 YEARS	50-64 YEARS	65 YEARS & OLDER
Tetanus, Diphtheria (Td)*	1 dose booster every 10 years		
Influenza	1 dose annually	1 dose annually	
Pneumococcal (polysaccharide)	1 dose		1 dose
Hepatitis B*	3 doses (0, 1–2, 4–6 months)		
Hepatitis A	2 doses (0, 6–12 months)		
Measles, Mumps, Rubella (MMR)*	1 dose if measles, mumps or rubella vaccination history is unreliable; 2 doses for persons with occupational or other indications		
Varicella*	2 doses (0, 4–8 weeks) for persons who are susceptible		
Meningococcal (polysaccharide)	1 dose		

* Covered by the Vaccine Injury Compensation Program. For information on how to file a claim, call **1-800-338-2382**. Please also visit **www.hrsa.osa.gov/vicp**. To file a claim for vaccine injury, write: U.S. Court of Federal Claims, 717 Madison Place, NW, Washington, DC 20005; Telephone 202 219 9657.

This schedule indicates the recommended age groups for routine administration of currently licensed vaccines for persons 19 years of age and older. Licensed combination vaccines may be used whenever any components of the combination are indicated and the vaccine's other components are not contraindicated. Providers should consult the manufacturers' package inserts for detailed recommendations.

APPROVED BY THE ADVISORY COMMITTEE ON IMMUNIZATION PRACTICES (ACIP) AND ACCEPTED BY THE AMERICAN COLLEGE OF OBSTETRICIANS AND GYNECOLOGISTS (ACOG) AND THE AMERICAN ACADEMY OF FAMILY PHYSICIANS (AAFP)

CDC National Immunization Hotline:
800-232-2522 ENGLISH • 800-232-0233 ESPAÑOL

Report all clinically significant post-vaccination reactions to the Vaccine Adverse Event Reporting System (VAERS). Reporting forms and instructions on filing a VAERS report are available by calling **1-800-822-7967** or from the VAERS website at **www.vaers.org**.

For additional information about the vaccines listed above and contraindications for immunization, please visit the National Immunization Program Website at: **www.cdc.gov/nip** or call the National Immunization Hotline, **1-800-232-2522** (English) or **1-800-232-0233** (Spanish).

Department of Health and Human Services
Centers for Disease Control and Prevention

Examples of Pediatric Developmental Milestones

Newborn: Eyes should fixate on objects
  Equal movements
  Responds to noises
  Fixes eyes on a changing stimulus
  Roots and sucks
1–3 months: Holds head up 45 degrees when prone
  Social smile
  Coos
  Uses limbs together
  Plays with hands and fingers
  Reaches for objects
  Supports self on forearms when on stomach
3–6 months: Lifts head up 90 degrees when prone
  Squeals
  Holds head erect when sitting
  Grasps object
  Follows object 180 degrees
  Rolls over to stomach and back by 6 months
  Can sit for few seconds without support
  Reaches for object
  Movements are more symmetric
  Most neonatal reflexes no longer present
6–9 months: Looks for fallen object
  Feeds self a cracker
  Sits alone
  Transfers object
  Stands holding on
  Palmar grasp developed
  Feeds self finger foods
  Birth weight doubles by 6 months
9–12 months: Pulls self to standing
  Stands holding on
  Plays peek-a-boo
  Birth weight triples
  Transfers object

9–12 months (Continued)
    Throws objects
    Has several teeth
    Rolls easily from back to stomach
    Sits alone steadily
    Hitches with backward movement
    Understands "No No"
    Speaks single words

12–18 months: Walks alone
    Indicates wants without crying
    Drinks from a cup
    Clumsily throws ball
    Climbs to get objects
    Removes some easily-removed clothes
    Understands simple instructions
    Can stack 3–4 blocks

18–24 months: Walks backward
    Feeds self with spoon
    Scribbles
    Walks stairs with help
    Finger paints
    Puts together large pieces of puzzle

2–3 years: Runs
    Climbs steps
    Draws a vertical line
    Solitary play
    Throws ball overhead
    Turns door handles
    Can use spoon to feed self
    Uses pronouns
    Uses simple sentences

3 years: Knows first name, age
    Uses plurals in speech
    Draws a circle
    Parallel or interactive play
    Dresses with help
    Pedals tricycle
    Builds using blocks
    Draws and paints

4 years: Knows last name
    Separates from parents
    Moves body smoothly
    Walks downstairs, both feet alternating

4 years (Continued)
  Interactive games
  Copies a square
  Can use scissors
5 years: Dresses alone
  Draws a square
  Follows commands
  Recognizes colors
  Jumps rope, hops, and skips
  Ties shoe laces
  Hand preference shown
6–8 years: Skips or rollerskates
  Prints numbers, letters
  Can tie a bow
  Defines six words
  Makes large letters
  Learns to pedal bicycle
  Changes from printing to cursive writing
8 + years: School grade is appropriate for age

Sample of Community Resources Available for Older People*

A. In-Home Services

Meals on Wheels
Chore services (housekeeping, yardwork)
Lifeline (emergency response systems)
Home health care, equipment, supplies, wheelchairs
Companion services (nonmedical)
Transportation (medical and social)
Insurance and Medicare information
Guardianship (limited or full)
Benefits counseling (representative payee, bill paying)
Adult protective services
In-home assessment (general, medical, mental)
Care coordination (case management)
Chronic disease-related agencies (arthritic, cancer, cardiovascular disease)
Hospice services

B. Residential Living

Retirement centers
Assisted living facilities
Personal care homes
Foster home care
Shared living
Life care settings such as a continuing care retirement community (from independent apartments to skilled nursing care)

---

* Refer to the area agency on aging in your community for specific phone numbers and other information.

C. Institutional and Health and/or Medical Resources

Nursing facilities (skilled nursing facilities, subacute care)

Hospitals (rehabilitation hospitals and units, skilled nursing units)

Long-term-care ombudsman program (advocacy for older persons)

Geriatric assessment and planning programs

Geriatric medical care (geriatrician and/or geriatric psychiatrist)

Gerontology specialists in medicine, nursing, social work, psychology

D. Family Support

Widowed persons' support groups

Family caregiver education classes

Support groups for family caregivers

As People Grow Older (APGO)

Children of Aging Parents support groups

Alzheimer's Association (information and support)

Adult day services

Respite care (short time)

Support groups for family caregivers

Sample Adult Physical Assessment Form with Guide

Name _____ Date _____

Age _____ Height _____ Weight _____ BMI _____

Waist Circumference _____

Frontal-Occipital Circumference _____

Vital Signs: T _____ P _____ R _____

BP: Sitting _____ Standing _____ Lying _____

Examination	Description*	Not Examined
Overall appearance		
Skin		
Head		
Eyes		
Ears		
Nose and sinuses		
Mouth and pharynx		

(Continued on following page)

(Continued)

Examination	Description*	Not Examined
Neck		
Thorax and lungs		
Breasts and axillae		
Heart and peripheral vascular system		
Abdomen		
Musculoskeletal system	.	
Genitourinary system and rectum		
Neurologic		
Mental status		
Laboratory and other pertinent data		

Source: Adapted from Physical Assessment Form 584. Harris School of Nursing, Texas Christian University, Fort Worth, TX, 2004, with permission.

Physical Assessment Guide

General Instructions

Use this guide for suggested descriptive terminology for documentation on the Sample Adult Physical Assessment Form.

Be specific, descriptive, and objective. Avoid such terms as "normal," "within normal limits," "good," "fair," and "O.K." Describe what you observe rather than make inferences or judgments.

Overall Appearance Inspection

Gender: Male/female.

General grooming: Clean? hair combed? makeup?

Position/posturing: Supine? prone? rigid? opisthotonos? erect? slumped?

Body size: Thin? overweight? obese? emaciated? flabby? weight proportionate to height? mesomorph? endomorph? ectomorph?

Facial expressions: Smiling? frowning? blank? apathetic?

Body language: Eye contact? no eye contact? arms folded over chest?

Other observations: Restless? fidgeting? lying quietly? listless? trembling? tense?

Skin Inspection and Palpation

Color and vascularity: Pink? tan? brown? dark brown? grayish? pasty? yellowish? flushed? jaundiced?

Turgor and mobility: Elastic? nonelastic? tenting? wrinkled? edematous? tight?

Temperature and moisture: Cold? cool? warm? hot? feverish? moist? dry? clammy? oily? sweating? diaphoresis?

Texture: Smooth? rough? fine? thick? coarse? scaly? puffy?

Nails: Clean? manicured? smooth? rough? dry? hard? brittle? splitting? cracking? angle of nail bed? clubbing? curved? flat? thick? yellowing? paronychia? *Nail beds and lunule:* Pale? pink? cyanotic? red? shape of lunule? blanching? spooning?

Body hair growth: Color? thick? thin? coarse? fine? location and distribution on body? hirsutism?

Skin integrity: Intact? not intact? *Lesions, birthmarks, moles, scars, and rashes* (describe shape, size, and location): Nevi? fissures? maculas? papules? pustules? nodules? bullae? cysts? carbuncles? wheals? erythema? excoriation? desquamation? abrasions? cherry angiomas? lentigines? purpura? keratoses? seborrheic keratoses? bruises? insect bites? crusts? warts? pimples? blackheads? bleeding? drainage? lacerations? scaly? ulcers? lichenification?

Head Inspection and Palpation

Shape: Round? oval? square? pointed? normocephalic?

Face: Oval? heart-shaped? pear? long? square? round? thin? high cheekbones? symmetrical?

Sensation (trigeminal—CN V): Sensation on three branches? clenched teeth?

Facial (CN VII): Facial expressions, smiles?

Hair: Color and growth: coarse? fine? thick? thin? sparse? alopecia? long? short? curly? straight? permed? glossy? shiny? greasy? dry? brittle? stringy? frizzy?

Condition of scalp: Clean? scaly? dandruff? rashes? sores? drainage?

Masses and lumps: Describe location and shape; measure size.

Eyes Inspection and Palpation

Eyebrows: Color and shape: Alignment? straight? curved? thick? thin? sparse? plucked? scaly?

Eyelashes: Long? short? curved? none? artificial?

Eyelids: Dark? swollen? inflamed? red? stye? infected? open and close simultaneously? ptosis? entropion? ectropion? lid lag? xanthomas?

Shape and appearance of eyes: Almond? rounded? squinty? prominent? exophthalmic? sunken? symmetrical? bright? clear? dull? tearing? discharge? (serous? purulent?) exotropia? esotropia? nystagmus? strabismus?

Sclera: White? cream? yellowish? jaundiced? injected? pterygium?

Conjunctivae: Pale pink? pink? red? inflamed? nodules? swelling?

Iris: Color and shape: Round? not round? coloboma? arcus senilis?

Cornea: Clear? milky? opaque? cloudy?

Pupils (oculomotor—CN III) [PERRLA]: Size and shape: (Measure in millimeters) Round? not round? (describe) *Equality:* Symmetrical? anisocoria? right larger than left? left larger than right? convergence? Reaction to light and accommodation? consensual reaction?

Extraocular movements (oculomotor), trochlear, (abducens—CN III, IV, VI): Intact?

Lacrimal glands: Tender? nontender? inflamed? swollen? tearing?

AIDS: Glasses? contact lenses? prosthesis?

Visual fields (optic—CN II): Intact?
Vision (optic—CN II): Reads newsprint? reports objects across room?

Ears Inspection and Palpation

Pinnae: Size and shape: large? small? in proportion to face? protruding? oval? large lobes? small lobes? symmetrical? right larger than left? left larger than right? pinnae irregular? color? skin intact? redness? swelling? tophi? cauliflower ear? furuncles? Darwin's tubercle?

Level in relation to eyes: Top of pinnae level with outer canthus of eyes? top of pinnae lower than outer canthus of eyes? top of pinnae higher than outer canthus of eyes? *Canal:* Clean? discharge? (serous? bloody? purulent?) nodules? inflammation? redness? foreign object? *Cilia:* Present/absent? *Cerumen:* Present/absent? color? consistency?

Tympanic membrane: Color? pearly white? injected? red? inflamed? discharge? cone of light? landmarks? scarring? bubbles? fluid level?

Hearing (auditory—CN VII): Right—present/absent? left—present/absent? hears watch tick? hears whisper? responds readily when spoken to? *Weber:* Lateralizes equally? to left/right side? *Rinne:* Air conduction > bone conduction 2:1? Hearing aid: Right/left.

Nose and Sinuses Inspection and Palpation

Size and shape: Long? short? large? small? in proportion to face? flat? broad? broad based? thick? enlarged? nares symmetrical/asymmetrical? pointed? swollen? bulbous? flaring of nostrils?

Septum: Midline? deviated right/left? perforated?

Nasal mucosa and turbinates: Pink? pale? bluish? red? dry? moist? discharge? (purulent? clear? watery? mucus?) cilia present/absent? rhinitis? epistaxis? polyps?

Patency of nares: (close each side and ask patient to breathe) Right—patent/partial obstruction/obstructed? left—patent/partial obstruction/obstructed?

Olfactory (CN I): Correctly identifies odors?

Sinuses: Tender? nontender? transillumination?

Mouth and Pharynx Inspection

Lips: Color: Pink? red? tan? pale? cyanotic? *Shape:* Thin? thick? enlarged? swollen? symmetrical/asymmetrical? drooping left side? drooping right side? *Condition:* Soft? smooth? dry? cracked? fissured? blisters? lesions? (describe)

Teeth: Color and condition: White? yellow? grayish? spotted? stained? darkened? pitting? notched? straight? crooked, protruding? separated? crowded? irregular? broken? notching? peglike? loose? dull? bright? edentulous? malocclusion? presence of dental caps or other appliances? *Caries and fillings:* Number and location? *Dental hygiene:* Clean? not clean?

Breath odor: Sweet? odorless? halitosis? musty? acetone? foul? fetid? odor of drugs or food? hot? sour? alcohol?

Gums: Pink? firm? swollen? bleeding? sensitive? gingivitis? hypertrophy? nodules? irritated? receding? moist? ulcerated? dry? shrunken? blistered? spongy?

Facial and glossopharyngeal (CN VII and IX): Identifies taste?

Tongue: Macroglossia? microglossia? glossitis? geographic? red? pink? pale? bluish? brownish? swollen? clean? thin? thick? fissured? raw? coated? moist? dry? cracked? glistening? papillae?

Hypoglossal (CN XII): Tongue movement: symmetry? lateral? fasciculation?

Mucosa: Color? leukoplakia? dry? moist? intact? not intact? masses? (describe size, shape, and location) chancre?

Palate: Moist? dry? color? intact? not intact?

Uvula: Color? midline? Remains at midline when saying "ah"? gag reflex present?

Pharynx: Color? petechia? injected? beefy? dysphagia?

Tonsils: Present/absent? cryptic? beefy? size 1+ to 4+?

Temporomandibular joint: Fully mobile? symmetrical? tenderness? crepitus?

Neck Inspection and Palpation

Appearance: Long? short? thick? thin? masses? (describe size and shape) symmetrical? not symmetrical?

Thyroid: Palpable? nodules? tender?

Trachea: Midline? deviated to right/left?

Lymph nodes: (Occipital, preauricular, postauricular, submental, submaxillary, tonsillar, anterior cervical, posterior cervical, superficial cervical, deep cervical, supraclavicular): Nonpalpable? tender? lymphadenopathy? shotty? hard? firm?

Thorax and Lungs Inspection, Palpation, Percussion, and Auscultation

Respirations: Rate? tachypnea, eupnea, bradypnea? apnea? orthopnea? labored? stertorous? *Rhythm:* Regular/irregular? inspiration time greater than expiration time? expiration time greater than inspiration time? spasmodic? gasping? orthopneic? deep? eupneic? shallow? flaring of nostrils with respirations? symmetrical/asymmetrical? right thorax greater than left? left thorax greater than right? ratio of AP diameter to lateral diameter between 1:2 and 5:7? ribs sloped downward at 45-degree angle? well-defined costal space? accessory muscles used? pigeon chest? funnel chest? barrel chest? abdominal or chest breather? skin intact? lesions? color? thin? muscular? flabby?

Posterior thorax: Tenderness? masses? *Respiratory excursion:* Symmetrical? asymmetrical? no respiratory movements on right/left? subcutaneous emphysema? crepitus? fremitus? estimation of level of diaphragm? spine alignment? tenderness? CVA tenderness? resonance? dull? hyperresonance? diaphragmatic excursion 3 to 5 cm? comparison of one side to the other? suprasternal notch located? costochondral junctions tender? chest wall stable? vocal fremitus?

Lung auscultation: Vesicular? bronchovesicular? bronchial? whispered pectoriloquy? adventitious sounds? rales? rhonchi? wheezes? crackles? rub? bronchophony? egophony?

Breasts and Axillae Inspection and Palpation

Breasts: Male? female? present/absent? color? large? small? well developed? firm? pendulous? flat? flabby? symmetrical/asymmetrical? dimpling? thickening? smooth? retraction? peau d'orange? venous pattern? tenderness? masses? (describe) gynecomastia?

Nipples: Present/absent? circular? symmetrical/asymmetrical? inverted? everted? pale? brown? rose? extra nipples? discharge? deviation? supernumerary?

Axillae: Shaved/unshaved? odor? masses or lumps? (describe size and shape)

Lymph nodes: (Lateral, central, subscapular, pectoral, epitrochlear) palpable? tender? shotty?

Heart and Peripheral Vascular Inspection, Percussion, Auscultation, and Palpation

Heart: Precordial bulge? abnormal palpations? Point of maximum intensity? thrills? heave or lift with pulsation? S_1 loudest at apex? S_2 loudest at base? S_3? S_4? splits? clicks? snap? rub? gallop? *Murmurs:* Systolic? diastolic? holosystolic? harsh? soft? blowing? rumbling? grading 1 through 6? high pitch? medium pitch? low pitch? radiating? pacemaker?

Carotid pulse: Note: Do not check both right and left carotid pulses simultaneously. Volume: Bounding? forceful? strong? full? weak? feeble? thready? symmetrical? right less than left? left less than right? *Rhythm:* Regular? irregular? symmetrical? asymmetrical? bruits present? absent?

Apical pulse: Record rate; tachycardia? bradycardia/pounding? forceful? weak? moderate? regular/irregular?

Peripheral pulses: (Do not count rate of these pulses except radial.) Record character, volume, rhythm, and symmetry of brachial, radial, femoral, popliteal, dorsalis pedis, and posterior tibial pulses. *Volume:* Full? strong? forceful? bounding? perceptible? imperceptible? weak? thready? symmetrical/asymmetrical? right greater than left? left greater than right? *Rhythm:* Regular? irregular? symmetrical? asymmetrical? *Symmetry:* Record as symmetrical, right greater than left or left greater than right? Pulse deficit, pulse pressure, BP in both arms, BP lying, sitting, and standing if applicable. Jugular venous distention? (Record centimeters above level of sternal angle.)

Abdomen Inspection, Auscultation, Percussion, Palpation

Contour: Irregular? protruding? enlarged? distended? scaphoid? concave? sunken? flabby? firm? flat? flaccid?

Skin: Color? intact? not intact? shiny? smooth? scars? lesions? (describe size, shape, and type of lesion) striae? umbilicus?

Bowel sounds: Present? absent? hyperactive? high-pitched tinkling? gurgles? borborygmus?

Percussion: Tympanic? dull? flat? (describe where) liver size 6 to 12 cm? splenic dullness 6th to 10th rib? ascites?

Palpation: Splenomegaly? hepatomegaly? organomegaly? masses? aortic pulse? diastasis recti? tenderness? bulges? lower pole of kidneys palpable? inguinal or femoral hernia? inguinal nodes? (describe)

Musculoskeletal Inspection and Palpation

Back: Shoulders level? right shoulder higher than left? left shoulder higher than right? alignment? lordosis? scoliosis? kyphosis? ankylosis?

Vertebral column alignment: Straight? lordosis? scoliosis? kyphosis?

Joints: Redness? swelling? deformity? (describe) crepitation? size? symmetry? subluxation? separation? bogginess? tenderness? pain? thickening? nodules? fluid? bulging? artificial?

Range of motion: Describe as full, limited, or fixed; estimate degree of limitation; assess range of motion of neck, shoulders, elbows, wrists, fingers, back, hips, knees, ankles, toes.

Extremities: Compare extremities with each other; describe color and symmetry. *Temperature:* Hot, warm, cool, cold, moist, clammy, dry. Muscle tone descriptors are firm, muscular, flabby, flaccid, atrophy? fasciculation? tremor?

Lower extremities: Symmetry? (Describe any variations from normal.) abrasions? bruises? swollen? edema? rashes/lesions? (describe) prosthesis? varicose veins?

Genitourinary and Rectum Inspection

Rectum: Hemorrhoids? inflammation? lesions? skin tags? fissures? excoriation? swelling? mucosal bulging? retrocele?

Female genitalia: Pubic hair distribution and color? nits? pediculosis? lesions? nodules? inflammation? swelling? pigmentation? dry? moist? shriveled, atrophied or full labia? discharge? (describe) odor? asymmetry? varicosities? uterine prolapse? smegma? rash?

Male genitalia: Pubic hair distribution and color? nits? pediculosis? circumcised? uncircumcised? phimosis? epispadias? hypospadias? smegma? priapism? varicocele? cryptorchism, hydrocele? swelling? redness? chancre? crusting? rash? discharge? (describe) edema? scrotal sack rugated? atrophy?

Neurologic

Describe tics, twitches, paresthesia, paralysis, coordination.

Gait: Balanced? shuffling? unsteady? ataxic? parkinsonian? swaying? scissor? spastic? waddling? staggering? faltering? swaying? slow? difficult? tottering? propulsive?

Accessory (CN XI): Shrugs shoulder? symmetry?

Reflexes: Report as present or absent.

Coordination: Report as to test done.

Cranial nerves: May be reported here.

Mental Status

Level of alertness: Alert? stuporous? semicomatose? comatose?

Orientation: Oriented to time, place, and person? confused? disoriented? If confused, check orientation as follows:

Time: Ask patient year, month, day, date.

Place: Ask patient's residence address, where she or he is now.

Person: Ask patient's name, birthday.

Memory: Recent memory: Give patient short series of numbers and ask patient to repeat those numbers later. *Long-term:* Ask patient to recall some event that happened several years ago.

Language and speech: Language spoken? *Speech:* Slurred? slow? rapid? difficulty forming words? aphasia?

Responsiveness: Responds appropriately to verbal stimuli? responds readily? slow to respond?

Seven Warning Signs of Cancer

See your health-care provider right away if you have:

- A sore that does not get better
- A nagging cough, or unusually hoarse voice
- Indigestion or problems with swallowing
- Changes in a wart or mole
- Unusual bleeding or discharge
- Thick spot or lump in breast or anywhere else
- Change in bowel or bladder habits

Source: Adapted from American Cancer Society, Inc, 1994.

APPENDIX M

Suggested Schedule of Health Screening for People Age 65 and Older with No Symptoms[1]

Exam	Both	Men	Women
1. Complete history and physical examination (including height and weight)	Annually		
2. BP; pulse <120/80 mm Hg; 50–100 beats per minute)	Every visit with physician		
3. Urinalysis	Periodic		
4. Breast physical examination (>age 40)			Annually
5. Mammogram (>age 40)[2]			Annually
6. Pelvic examination (>age 40)[3]			Annually
7. Pap smear[3] (>age 40)			Every 24 months (every 12 months if high risk)
8. Digital rectal examination (>age 40)[2]	Annually	Check prostate annually	
9. Prostate-specific antigen (PSA) blood test (>age 50)[2]		Annually	
10. Fecal occult blood test (>age 50)[2]	Annually		
11. Dental and oral examination	Semiannually		
12. Vision exam (glaucoma,[6] cataracts[4])	Annually		

(Continued on next page)

(Continued)

Exam	Both	Men	Women
13. Hearing examination	Periodic		
14. Total skin self-examination	Monthly		
15. Breast self-examination (BSE)			Monthly
16. Testicular self-examination (TSE)		Monthly	
17. Influenza vaccination[2]	Annually (October/November best, can be later)		
18. Pneumococcal vaccination[4]	Once only (more often if high risk; some physicians recommend every 5–6 years)		
19. Tetanus-diphtheria booster (Td)	Every 10 years after first series		
20. Hepatitis B vaccination[4,5]	Three doses—once only		
21. Tuberculosis skin test (PPD)[5]	As needed (e.g., living in nursing facility)		
22. Cholesterol[4–6] <200 mg/dL, HDL >35 mg/dL, LDL <130 mg/dL	Every 6 months–1 year if > 200 mg/dL		
23. Thyroid function test	Annually		
24. Blood sugar (60–110 mg/dL)[7]	Periodic		
25. Hematocrit/hemoglobin	Periodic		
26. Sigmoidoscopy or barium enema (>age 50)[8,9]	Every 2–4 years		
27. Colonoscopy or barium enema[9,10]	Every 2–10 years		
28. Electrocardiogram (ECG)[5,6]	Periodic		

Exam	Both	Men	Women
29. Endometrial tissue biopsy[5]			At menopause
30. Pelvic sonogram[5]			Periodic
31. Bone mineral density (BMD) measurements to detect osteoporosis (>age 50)[3]			At least once and periodic based on results
32. Chest x-ray	Not routinely recommended		

[1]*These suggestions assume that the persons are healthy and not high risk (except where indicated) for any major diseases because of family history or other factors. Individual decisions must be made by the person and physician. Numerical norms may vary based on different references.*

[2] *Covered by Medicare every 12 months.*

[3] *Covered by Medicare once every 2 years on an individual high-risk basis. Every year if high risk.*

[4] *Covered by Medicare.*

[5] *If high risk.*

[6] *Based on family history.*

[7] *May be higher without a diagnosis of diabetes in older adults.*

[8] *Covered by Medicare every 4 years.*

[9] *Covered by Medicare every 2 years if high risk.*

[10] *Covered by Medicare every 10 years if not high risk.*

References

American Lung Association, State Office, August 10, 1994.

Barbacia, JS: Prevention. In Longergan, ET: Geriatrics. Appleton and Lange, Stamford, CT, 1996.

Crowley, SL: New Budget Finances Preventive Care. AARP Bulletin, 38(9):6, October 1997.

Cancer Facts and Figures—1994. American Cancer Society, Atlanta, GA 1994.

Goldberg, T, and Chavm, S: Preventive Medicine and Screening in Older Adults. J Am Geriatr Soc 45:344–354, 1997.

Ham, RJ, and Sloane, PD: Primary Care Geriatrics: A Case-based Approach, ed 2. St Louis, Mosby, 1992.

Knebl, JA: Chief, Division of Geriatrics, University of North Texas Health Science Center at Fort Worth. Personal communication, 1994; March 18, 1999.

National Institute on Aging: Bound for Good Health, A Collection of Seventh Report of the Joint National Committee on Prevention,

Age Pages. Author, Washington, DC Detection, Evaluation, and Treatment of High Blood Pressure, June 3, 2003 http://www.american heart.org/presenter:html?identifier=3011728.

U.S. Department of Health and Human Services: Centers for Medicare and Medicaid Services Medicare and You 2005. Pub. No. CMS. 10050, Baltimore, MD, 2003.

Food Guide Pyramid

A Guide to Daily Food Choices

The Food Guide Pyramid is not a prescription but a general guide of what to eat each day. It suggests eating a variety of foods to get the nutrients you need and also eating the right amounts of each food group to maintain a healthy weight. The Food Guide Pyramid emphasizes foods from the five food groups shown in the sections of the pyramid. None of these groups is more important than another; a healthy diet needs all of the nonfat groups. The Food Guide Pyramid has been modified for people age 70 and older.

Original Food Guide Pyramid

Fats, oils, & sweets
Use sparingly

Milk, yogurt, & cheese group
2-3 servings

Meat, poultry, fish, dry beans, eggs, & nuts group
2-3 servings

Vegetable group
3-5 servings

Fruit group
2-4 servings

Bread, cereal, rice, & pasta group
6-11 servings

Source: U.S. Departments of Agriculture and Health and Human Services.

Food Guide Pyramid for Older Adults

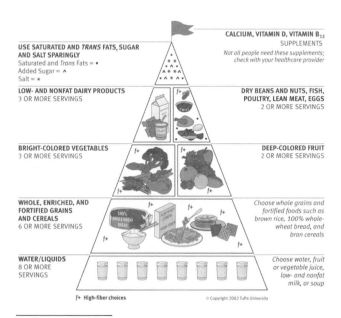

CALCIUM, VITAMIN D, VITAMIN B$_{12}$
SUPPLEMENTS
*Not all people need these supplements;
check with your healthcare provider*

USE SATURATED AND *TRANS* FATS, SUGAR
AND SALT SPARINGLY
Saturated and *Trans* Fats = •
Added Sugar = ∧
Salt = *

LOW- AND NONFAT DAIRY PRODUCTS
3 OR MORE SERVINGS

DRY BEANS AND NUTS, FISH,
POULTRY, LEAN MEAT, EGGS
2 OR MORE SERVINGS

BRIGHT-COLORED VEGETABLES
3 OR MORE SERVINGS

DEEP-COLORED FRUIT
2 OR MORE SERVINGS

WHOLE, ENRICHED, AND
FORTIFIED GRAINS
AND CEREALS
6 OR MORE SERVINGS

*Choose whole grains and
fortified foods such as
brown rice, 100% whole-
wheat bread, and
bran cereals*

WATER/LIQUIDS
8 OR MORE
SERVINGS

*Choose water, fruit
or vegetable juice,
low- and nonfat
milk, or soup*

f+ High-fiber choices

© Copyright 2002 Tufts University

Source: Russell, R.M. Rasmussen, H. and Lichtenstein, A.H.: Modified food
guide pyramid for people over seventy years of age. Journal of Nutrition
129:752© Tufts University, with permission.

APPENDIX O

Healthy Weight Charts and Body Mass Index (BMI)

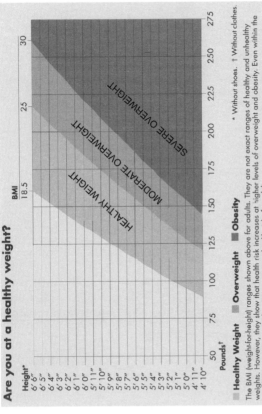

Are you at a healthy weight?

The BMI (weigh-for-height) ranges shown above are for adults. They are not exact ranges of healthy and unhealthy weights. However, they show that health risk increases at higher levels of overweight and obesity. Even within the healthy BMI range, weight gains can carry health risks for adults.

■ Healthy Weight ■ Overweight ■ Obesity

* Without shoes. † Without clothes.

* Without Shoes
** Without Clothes

Source: *Report of the Dietary Guidelines Advisory Committee on the Dietary Guidelines for Americans, 2000.* Available at: http://www.ars.usda.gov/dgac/ dgacguideexp.pdf. Accessed February 23, 2000.

2 to 20 years: Girls
Body mass index-for-age percentiles

NAME

RECORD #

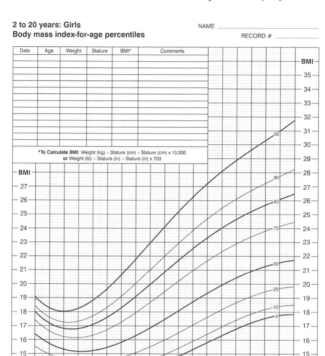

*To Calculate BMI: Weight (kg) ÷ Stature (cm) ÷ Stature (cm) x 10,000
or Weight (lb) ÷ Stature (in) ÷ Stature (in) x 703*

Published May 30, 2000 (modified 10/16/00).
SOURCE: Developed by the National Center for Health Statistics in collaboration with
the National Center for Chronic Disease Prevention and Health Promotion (2000).
http://www.cdc.gov/growthcharts

Published May 30, 2000 (modified 10/16/00).
Source: Developed by the National Center for Health Statistics in collaboration
with the National Center for Chronic Disease Prevention and Health Promotion
(2000). http://www.cdc.gov/growthcharts

2 to 20 years: Boys
Body mass index-for-age percentiles

NAME _____

RECORD # _____

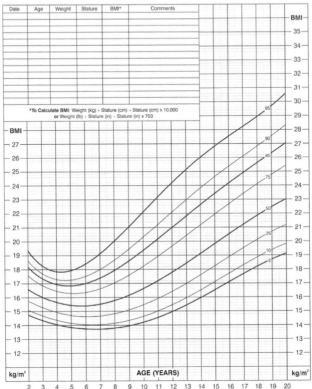

Date	Age	Weight	Stature	BMI*	Comments

*To Calculate BMI: Weight (kg) ÷ Stature (cm) ÷ Stature (cm) x 10,000
or Weight (lb) ÷ Stature (in) ÷ Stature (in) x 703

AGE (YEARS)

Published May 30, 2000 (modified 10/16/00).
SOURCE: Developed by the National Center for Health Statistics in collaboration with
the National Center for Chronic Disease Prevention and Health Promotion (2000).
http://www.cdc.gov/growthcharts

Published May 30, 2000 (modified 10/16/00).
Source: Developed by the National Center for Health Statistics in collaboration
with the National Center for Chronic Disease Prevention and Health Promotion
(2000). http://www.cdc.gov/growthcharts

HEIGHT \ WEIGHT	100	105	110	115	120	125	130	135	140	145	150	155	160	165	170	175	180	185	190	195	200	205	210	215	220
5'0"	20	21	21	22	23	24	25	26	27	28	29	30	31	32	33	34	35	36	37	38	39	40	41	42	43
5'1"	19	20	21	22	23	24	25	26	26	27	28	29	30	31	32	33	34	35	36	37	38	39	40	41	42
5'2"	18	19	20	21	22	23	24	25	26	27	27	28	29	30	31	32	33	34	35	36	37	37	38	39	40
5'3"	18	19	19	20	21	22	23	24	25	26	27	27	28	29	30	31	32	33	34	35	35	36	37	38	39
5'4"	17	18	19	20	21	21	22	23	24	25	26	27	27	28	29	30	31	32	33	33	34	35	36	37	38
5'5"	17	17	18	19	20	21	22	22	23	24	25	26	27	27	28	29	30	31	32	32	33	34	35	36	37
5'6"	16	17	18	19	19	20	21	22	23	23	24	25	26	27	27	28	29	30	31	31	32	33	34	35	36
5'7"	16	16	17	18	19	20	20	21	22	23	23	24	25	26	27	27	28	29	30	31	31	32	33	34	34
5'8"	15	16	17	17	18	19	20	21	21	22	23	24	24	25	26	27	27	28	29	30	30	31	32	33	33
5'9"	15	16	16	17	18	18	19	20	21	21	22	23	24	24	25	26	27	27	28	29	30	30	31	32	32
5'10"	14	15	16	16	17	18	19	19	20	21	22	22	23	24	24	25	26	27	27	28	29	29	30	31	32
5'11"	14	15	15	16	17	17	18	19	20	20	21	22	22	23	24	24	25	26	26	27	28	29	29	30	31
6'0"	14	14	15	16	16	17	18	18	19	20	20	21	22	22	23	24	24	25	26	26	27	28	28	29	30
6'1"	13	14	15	15	16	16	17	18	18	19	20	20	21	22	22	23	24	24	25	26	26	27	28	28	29
6'2"	13	13	14	15	15	16	17	17	18	19	19	20	21	21	22	22	23	24	24	25	26	26	27	28	28
6'3"	12	13	14	14	15	16	16	17	17	18	19	19	20	21	21	22	22	23	24	24	25	26	26	27	27
6'4"	12	13	13	14	15	15	16	16	17	18	18	19	19	20	21	21	22	23	23	24	24	25	26	26	27

SOURCES: Shape Up America; National Institutes of Health

The BMI score means the following: Underweight Below 18.5; Normal 18.5–24.9; Overweight 25.0–29.9; Obesity 30.0–39.9; Extreme obesity ≥40

Source: National Heart, Lung, and Blood Institute Obesity Education Initiative. Expert Panel. Clinical guidelines on the identification, evaluation and treatment of overweight and obesity in adults. Available at:http://www.nhlbi.nih.gov. Accessed November 8, 1999.

Physical Signs of Malnutrition and Deficiency State

■ Infants and Children

Lack of subcutaneous fat
Wrinkling of skin on light stroking
Poor muscle tone
Pallor
Rough skin (toad skin)
Hemorrhage of newborn, vitamin K deficiency
Bad posture
Nasal area red and greasy
Sores at angles of mouth, cheilosis
Rapid heartbeat
Red tongue
Square head, wrists enlarged, rib beading
Vincent's angina, thrush
Serious dental abnormalities
Corneal and conjunctival changes

■ Adolescents and Adults

Nasolabial sebaceous plugs
Sores at corners of mouth, cheilosis
Vincent's angina
Minimal changes in tongue color or texture
Red swollen lingual papillac
Glossitis
Papillary atrophy of tongue
Stomatitis
Spongy, bleeding gums
Muscle tenderness in extremities
Hyperesthesia of skin
Bilateral symmetrical dermatitis
Purpura
Dermatitis: Facial butterfly, perineal, scrotal, vulval
Thickening and pigmentation of skin over bony prominences
Nonspecific vaginitis
Follicular hyperkeratosis of extensor surfaces of extremities
Rachitic chest deformity
Anemia not responding to iron

Source: Adapted from Committee on Medical Nutrition, National Research Council.

Poor muscle tone
Loss of vibratory sensation
Increase or decrease of tendon reflexes

Fatigue of visual accommodation
Vascularization of cornea
Conjunctival changes

Older Adults

Progressive weight loss
Reduced appetite
Prominence of the bony skeleton
Muscle wasting
Glossitis
Mouth sores
Cracked lips
Brittle hair and nails
Dry rough skin
Nonhealing wounds

Sunken eyes
Pale sclerae
Peripheral edema
Lack of energy or generalized weakness
Blunted mental status
Decreased deep tendon reflexes
Decreased vibratory sense
Bleeding gums and poor dentition

A Guide for Healthy Aging

Note: Check with your private physician before you make any major changes in your health practices, activities, or lifestyle

Good Nutrition

- Eat a variety of foods in moderation.
- Eat less but more frequently.
- Decrease calories, fat, sugar, salt, cholesterol.
- Increase fiber, grains, fruits, vegetables (especially green and yellow).
- Drink 8—8 ounces of fluid daily (decrease caffeine).
- Take one good multivitamin/mineral supplement daily, especially vitamins B, C, E, and calcium but not excessive amounts of any one vitamin.

Exercise

- Benefits: Decreases blood pressure, weight, cholesterol, stress, and depression; increases relaxation, attitude, sleep, mood, energy, and calcium in bones; maintains muscle function; strengthens heart and lungs.
- Amount: 30 minutes three to five times a week as a minimum.
- Type: Walking and swimming are the best; consistency is more important than how strenuous it is.

Immunizations

- Influenza every year (October-November)
- Pneumococcal (once only; more often if recommended by physician)

- Hepatitis B (3 doses—once only)
- Tetanus/diphtheria (Td) booster (every 10 years)

Health Screening

- Annual physical examination with your health-care provider.
- Exact screening tests will be based on age, gender, personal risk factors based on family history and lifestyle, physician recommendations, and patient preferences.
- Ask the physician about a prostate-specific antigen test—PSA (men), mammogram, thyroid, and bone mineral density (BMD) (women), and eye and colon exams (both men and women).
- Keep your own record of medical tests, treatments, and physician office visits.

Medications

- Take as few as needed for chronic diseases and take for a limited time frame for acute illnesses.
- Ask your physician about taking a low-dose (81 mg) aspirin daily (contraindicated if taking blood-thinning medications).

Do Not Smoke

If You Drink Moderation Is Important

Keep as Active as Possible, Both Physically and Mentally

- Maintain contact with family members and friends.
- Stay active in the community (work, recreation, volunteer).
- Do what you enjoy, not what others expect of you—everyone is different.
- Keep a positive attitude.

Recommended Dietary Nutrients and Sources

Water-Soluble Vitamins	Important Food Sources	Role in the Body
Ascorbic acid (vitamin C)	Citrus fruits, cantaloupe, tomatoes, strawberries, sweet peppers, cabbage, potatoes, broccoli, parsley	Promotes healing of wounds/fractures Maintains integrity of capillaries Aids tooth and bone formation Protects folic acid Increases iron absorption Helps form collagen
Thiamin (vitamin B_1)	Liver, pork, chicken, fish, beef, whole grains, wheat germ, dried yeast, enriched cereal products, nuts, and lentils	Metabolizes carbohydrates for energy Provides function of nerve cell membranes
Riboflavin (vitamin B_2)	Milk, liver, meat, fish, eggs, enriched cereal products, green leafy vegetables	Metabolizes carbohydrates for energy Provides function of nerve cell membranes
Niacin	Liver, poultry, meat, fish, eggs, whole grains, enriched cereal products, peanuts, and peanut butter	Metabolizes carbohydrates for energy
Pyridoxine (vitamin B_6)	Organ meats, pork, meat poultry, fish, legumes, seeds, whole grains	Metabolizes protein, converts tryptophan to niacin, maintains integrity of central nervous system, synthesizes hemoglobin
Vitamin B_{12} (cyanocobalamin)	Animal foods only—liver, meat, salt-water fish, oysters, eggs, milk	Essential for red blood cell maturation and normal function of all cells
Folate	Green leafy vegetables, liver, beef, fish, dry beans, lentils, whole grains	Essential for DNA synthesis and synthesis/maturation of red blood cells
Pantothenic acid	Animal sources (esp. organ meats, egg yolk, and meat), whole grains, legumes, yeast	Active in metabolism of carbohydrates, proteins, fats for energy; formation of hormones, hemoglobin, and neurochemicals

	Important Food Sources	Role in the Body
biotin	Organ meats, egg yolk, legumes, nuts	Synthesizes fatty acids, metabolizes carbohydrates for energy
Fat-Soluble Vitamins	**Important Food Sources**	**Role in the Body**
Vitamin A (retinol, beta carotene)	Milk, butter, fortified margarine, whole milk, cheese, liver, egg yolk, green leafy and stem vegetables, yellow fruits and vegetables (carotene); broccoli, carrots, apricots and cantaloupe	Maintains normal vision in dim light, healthy skin, and mucous membranes; essential for normal skeletal and tooth development
Vitamin D (calciferol)	Exposure to sunlight, fortified foods, fish liver oils	Maintains blood calcium and phosphorus levels necessary for bone development
Vitamin E (tocopherol)	Vegetable oils, whole grains, wheat germ, leafy vegetables, egg yolk, legumes, nuts, sunflower seeds	Protects integrity of normal cell membranes, assists in prevention of hemolysis of red blood cells, protects vitamin A, and acts as an antioxidant
Vitamin K	Spinach, lettuce, kale, cauliflower, egg yolk, liver	Produces prothrombin in normal blood clotting
Minerals	**Important Food Sources**	**Role in the Body**
Calcium	Milk, hard cheeses, yogurt, ice cream, cottage cheese, turnip and mustard greens, collards, kale, broccoli	Maintains strength of bones and teeth; involved with nerve transmission, muscle contraction/relaxation, blood clotting

(Continued on following page)

(Continued)

Minerals	Important Food Sources	Role in the Body
Phosphorus	Milk and milk products, meat, poultry, fish and eggs, whole grain cereals and flours, nuts and legumes	Essential for structure of bones and teeth; release of stored energy; structure of RNA/DNA; metabolism of carbohydrates, fats, protein
Magnesium	Whole grain breads and cereals, soybeans, nuts, dry beans and peas, green leafy vegetables	Active in production of energy; bone metabolism; maintenance of muscles and nerve tissue
Sodium	Use of salt at the table and in cooking, processed foods, milk, eggs, meat, poultry, fish, smoked meats, olives, pickles, soy sauce	Maintains osmotic pressure and water balance, normal nerve cell activity, contraction of muscles, permeability of cell membrane
Potassium	Meats, poultry, fish, fruits and vegetables (esp. bananas, potatoes, tomatoes, citrus fruits), whole grain cereals	Maintains osmotic pressure and water balance, transmission of nerve impulse, and contraction of muscles
Chloride	Use of salt at the table/in cooking	Regulates osmotic pressure, water balance, acid-base balance of extracellular fluid, component of hydrochloric acid

Trace Elements	Important Food Sources	Role in the Body
Iron	Liver, meat, fish and poultry, whole grains, enriched cereals, legumes, green leafy vegetables, eggs, dried fruits	Essential for hemoglobin and myoglobin formation—and supply of oxygen to cells

Nutrient	Sources	Function
Zinc	Animal products (esp. liver and oysters), beef, lamb, pork, whole grain cereals, legumes, peanuts, peanut butter	Necessary for wound healing, synthesis of proteins, mobilization of vitamin A from liver, immune function, and growth/development of genital organs
Copper	Organ meats, shellfish (esp. oysters and crab), whole grain cereals, hickory and brazil nuts, sesame and sunflower seeds, legumes	Essential for formation of red blood cells and use of iron, production of energy, protects cell against oxidative damage, synthesis of connective tissue
Iodine	Iodized salt used at the table and in cooking	Component of thyroid hormones, influences physical and mental growth, maintains nerve/muscle tissue, circulatory activity, metabolism of all nutrients
Fluoride	Fluoridated water, seafood	Increases calcium deposition and strengthens bone tissue
Chromium Manganese Molybdenum Selenium Nickel Silicon Vanadium	Present in very small amounts in plant foods (whole grains, dried beans, peas, nuts, seeds, fresh fruits, vegetables), animal foods	Essential as component of enzymes and hormones

Source: Adapted from American Dietetic Association—Complete Food and Nutrition Guide, ed 2, 2002; and Morrison's Manual of Clinical Nutrition Management, 2003.

Glasgow Coma Scale

Eye Opening	Points	Best Verbal Response	Points	Best Motor Response	Points
Spontaneous: Indicates arousal mechanisms in brainstem are active.	4	*Oriented:* Patient knows who and where he is, and the year, season, and month.	5	*Obeys commands:* Do not class a grasp reflex or change in posture as a response.	6
To sound: Eyes open to any sound stimulus.	3	*Confused:* Responses to questions indicate varying degrees of confusion and disorientation.	4	*Localized:* Moves a limb to attempt to remove stimulus	5
To pain: Apply stimulus to limbs, not to face.	2	*Inappropriate:* Speech is intelligible, but sustained conversation is not possible.	3	*Flexor normal:* Entire shoulder or arm is flexed in response to painful stimuli.	4
Never	1	*Incomprehensible:* Patient makes unintelligible sounds such as moans and groans.	2	*Flexion abnormal:* Slow stereotyped assumption of decorticate rigidity posture in response to painful stimuli.	3
		None	1	*Extension:* Abnormal with adduction and internal rotations of the shoulder and pronation of the forearm.	2
				None: Be certain that a lack of response is not attributable to a spinal cord injury.	1

Note: This scale, originally described in 1974 and further discussed in 1979 by Teasdale and his associates, is widely used in assessing head injury patients, both at the time of the injury and as the patient is observed. The score is recorded every 2 to 3 days.
Source: Adapted from Teasdale, G, and Jennett, B: Lancet II, 1974, p 81, and Teasdale, G, et al: Acta Neurochirurgica (suppl) 28, 1979, pp 13–16.

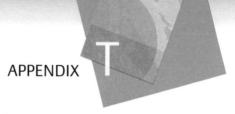

APPENDIX T

Client Positions

POSITIONS

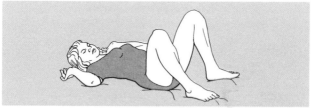

DORSAL RECUMBENT POSITION

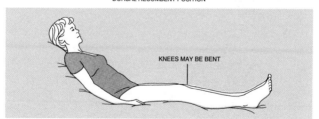

KNEES MAY BE BENT

FOWLER'S POSITION

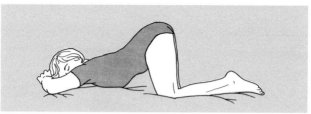

KNEE-CHEST OR GENUPECTORAL POSITION

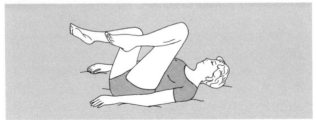

LITHOTOMY OR DORSOSACRAL POSITION

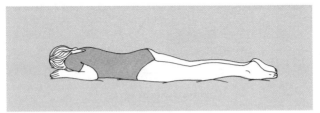

PRONE POSITION

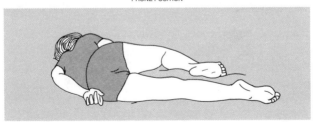

SIMS' POSITION

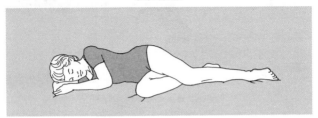

RIGHT LATERAL RECUMBENT POSITION

Source: Taber's, 2001, ed 19, pp 1714–1715, with permission.

Conversion Rules

To convert units of one system into the other, multiply the number of units in column I by the equivalent factor opposite that unit in column II.

WEIGHT

I		II
1 milligram	–	0.015432 grain
1 gram	–	15.432 grains
1 gram	–	0.25720 apothecaries' dram
1 gram	–	0.03527 avoirdupois ounce
1 gram	–	0.03215 apothecaries' or troy ounce
1 kilogram	–	35.274 avoirdupois ounces
1 kilogram	–	32.151 apothecaries' or troy ounces
1 kilogram	–	2.2046 avoirdupois pounds
1 grain	–	64.7989 milligrams
1 grain	–	0.0648 gram
1 apothecaries' dram	–	3.8879 grams
1 avoirdupois ounce	–	28.3495 grams
1 apothecaries' or troy ounce	–	31.1035 grams
1 avoirdupois pound	–	453.5924 grams

VOLUME (AIR OR GAS)

I		II
1 cubic centimeter	–	0.06102 cubic inch
1 cubic meter	–	35.314 cubic feet
1 cubic meter	–	1.3079 cubic yard
1 cubic inch	–	16.3872 cubic centimeters
1 cubic foot	–	0.02832 cubic meter

(Continued on following page)

(Continued)

CAPACITY (FLUID OR LIQUID)

I		II
1 milliliter	–	16.23 minim
1 milliliter	–	0.2705 fluidram
1 milliliter	–	0.0338 fluidounce
1 liter	–	33.8148 fluidounces
1 liter	–	2.1134 pints
1 liter	–	1.0567 quarts
1 liter	–	0.2642 gallon
1 fluidram	–	3.697 milliliters
1 fluidounce	–	29.573 milliliters
1 pint	–	473.1765 milliliters
1 quart	–	946.353 milliliters
1 gallon	–	3.785 liters

▓ To Convert Celsius or Centigrade Degrees to Fahrenheit Degrees

Multiply the number of Celsius degrees by 9/5 and add 32 to the result.
Example: $55°C \times 9/5 = 99 + 32 = 131°F$

▓ To Convert Fahrenheit Degrees to Celsius or Centigrade Degrees

Subtract 32 from the number of Fahrenheit degrees and multiply the difference by 5/9.
Example: $243°F - 32 = 211 \times 5/9 = 117.2°C$

Source: Adapted from Taber's Cyclopedic Medical Dictionary, ed 19, 2001; pp 703, 1714–1715 with permission.

APPENDIX V

Weights and Measures

Apothecaries' Weight

20 grains = 1 scruple
8 grains = 1 ounce

3 scruples = 1 dram
12 ounces = 1 pound

Avoirdupois Weight

27.343 grains = 1 dram
16 ounces = 1 pound
2000 pounds = 1 short ton
1 ounce troy = 480 grains
1 pound troy = 5760 grains

16 drams = 1 ounce
100 pounds = 1 hundredweight
2240 pounds = 1 long ton
1 ounce avoirdupois = 437.5 grains
1 pound avoirdupois = 7000 grains

Circular Measure

60 seconds = 1 minute
90 degrees = 1 quadrant

60 minutes = 1 degree
4 quadrants = 360 degrees = circle

Cubic Measure

1728 cubic inches = 1 cubic foot
2150.42 cubic inches = 1 standard bushel
1 cubic foot = about four-fifths of a bushel

27 cubic feet = 1 cubic yard
268.8 cubic inches = 1 dry (U.S.) gallon
128 cubic feet = 1 cord (wood)

Dry Measure

2 pints = 1 quart

8 quarts = 1 peck

4 pecks = 1 bushel

Liquid Measure

16 ounces = 1 pint
1000 milliliters = 1 liter
4 gills = 1 pint

4 quarts = 1 gallon
31.5 gallons = 1 barrel (U.S.)
2 pints = 1 quart

2 barrels = 1 hogshead (U.S.)
1 quart = 946.35 milliliters
1 liter = 1.0566 quart

Barrels and hogsheads vary in size. A U.S. gallon is equal to 0.8327 British gallon; therefore, a British gallon is equal to 1.201 U.S. gallon. 1 liter is equal to 1.0567 quart.

Linear Measure

1 inch = 2.54 centimeters
12 inches = 1 foot
1 statute mile = 5280 feet

40 rods = 1 furlong
3 feet = 1 yard
3 statute miles = 1 statute league

8 furlongs = 1 statute mile
5.5 yards = 1 rod
1 nautical mile = 6076.042 feet

Troy Weight

24 grains = 1 pennyweight
Used for weighing gold, silver, and jewels

20 pennyweights = 1 ounce

12 ounces = 1 pound

(Continued on following page)

Household Measures* and Weights

Approximate Equivalents:
60 drops

= 1 teaspoonful = 5 mL = 60 minims = 60 grains = 1 dram = 1/8 ounce

1 teaspoon = 1/8 fluid ounce; 1 dram

3 teaspoons = 1 tablespoon   16 tablespoons (liquid) = 1 cup

1 tablespoon = 1/2 fluid ounce; 4 drams   12 tablespoons (dry) = 1 cup

1 tumbler or glass = 8 fluid ounces; 1/2 pint   1 cup = 8 fluid ounces

*Household measures are not precise. For instance, a household teaspoon will hold from 3 to 5 mL of liquid substances. Therefore, do not substitute household equivalents for medication prescribed by the physician.

Source: Taber's Cyclopedic Medical Dictionary, ed 19. FA Davis, Philadelphia, 2001, p 2486, with permission.

(Continued)

APPENDIX W

Fahrenheit and Celsius Scales

Thermometric Equivalents (Celsius and Fahrenheit)

C°	F°	C°	F°	C°	F°	C°	F°
0	32	27	80.6	54	129.2	81	177.8
1	33.8	28	82.4	55	131	82	179.6
2	35.6	29	84.2	56	132.8	83	181.4
3	37.4	30	86.0	57	134.6	84	183.2
4	39.2	31	87.8	58	136.4	85	185
5	41	32	89.6	59	138.2	86	186.8
6	42.8	33	91.4	60	140	87	188.6
7	44.6	34	93.2	61	141.8	88	190.4
8	46.4	35	95	62	143.6	89	192.2
9	48.2	36	96.8	63	145.4	90	194
10	50	37	98.6	64	147.2	91	195.8
11	51.8	38	100.4	65	149	92	197.6
12	53.6	39	102.2	66	150.8	93	199.4
13	55.4	40	104	67	152.6	94	201.2
14	57.2	41	105.8	68	154.4	95	203
15	59	42	107.6	69	156.2	96	204.8
16	60.8	43	109.4	70	158	97	206.6
17	62.6	44	111.2	71	159.8	98	208.4
18	64.4	45	113	72	161.6	99	210.2
19	66.2	46	114.8	73	163.4	100	212
20	68	47	116.6	74	165.2		
21	69.8	48	118.4	75	167		
22	71.6	49	120.2	76	168.8		
23	73.4	50	122	77	170.6		
24	75.2	51	123.8	78	172.4		
25	77	52	125.6	79	174.2		
26	78.8	53	127.4	80	176		

Source: Taber's Cyclopedic Medical Dictionary, ed 19. FA Davis, Philadelphia. 2001, p 771, with permission.

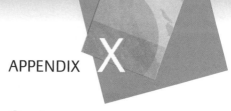

Medication Card

MEDICATION CARD
NAME _____
ADDRESS _____ _____
DATE OF BIRTH _____
DATE CARD FILLED OUT _____
EMERGENCY CONTACT PHONE _____
HOSPITAL PREFERRED _____
PHYSICIAN _____   PHONE _____
MAJOR ILLNESSES
MEDICATION ALLERGIES

Medication card. **Source:** Harris School of Nursing, Texas Christian University, 2004. Used with permission.

PRESCRIPTION MEDICATIONS		
NAME	**DOSE**	**TIMES TAKEN**

OVER-THE-COUNTER MEDICATIONS		
(vitamins, herbs, supplements)		

TCU **TAKE CARE OF YOUR HEALTH**
HARRIS SCHOOL OF NURSING
TEXAS CHRISTIAN UNIVERSITY

It is recommended that patients carry a completed medication card in their purse, pocket, or billfold at all times, so that they will have this essential information when visiting a physician's office or an emergency department.

APPENDIX Y

Newborn Physical Assessment Guide

This is a guide to assist you in the assessment of a newborn. The first term in the category is usually the normal expected finding, *italicized words* are variations of normal or abnormal findings, *<u>italicized and underlined</u>* are gestational age assessment findings.

💾 General Information

(You may obtain this information from mother's and baby's charts) Length of prenatal care? high-risk factors? date of birth? type of delivery? pregnancy/delivery complications? birth length? Apgar scores? gestation (weeks)? age (days/hours)? today's weight? birth weight?

Skin Inspection and Palpation

Color and vascularity: Ethnic grouping? pink? acrocyanosis? Mongolian spots? Milia? *central cyanosis? pale? plethoric? mottled? jaundice? abrasions? birthmarks? meconium staining? ecchymosis? lacerations? petechiae? <u>opacity?</u>*
Turgor: Elastic? tenting?
Temperature and moisture: Dry? moist?
Texture and integrity: Smooth and intact? *eruptions? not intact? lesions? pustules? rash? skin tags? vesicles? <u>lanugo? peeling? dry?</u>*
Nails: Soft? cover entire nail bed? beyond fingertips? meconium staining?

Head Inspection and Palpation

Shape: Symmetrical without molding? *caput? asymmetrical? molding? cephalhematoma? forceps marks?*

Source: Harris School of Nursing, Texas Christian University. Fort Worth. Tex, 2004, with permission.

Fontanel: Flat? *sunken? full? bulging? tense? sagittal suture— smooth without ridges? overriding?*
Face: Symmetrical? *asymmetrical?*

Eyes Inspection

Sclera: Clear? bluish-white? blink reflex? *jaundice? tearing?*
Conjunctiva: Clear? *jaundice? hemorrhage?*
Pupils: Reactions to light? PERRLA?
Retina: Red reflex present?
Eyelids: Movements? *prominent epicanthal folds? placement? edema?*
Eye movements: Present?

Ears Inspection and Palpation

Pinnae: Position/placement: aligned with eyes? skin tags? preauricular sinus? *curvature? cartilage development? recoil?*

Nose Inspection and Palpation

Symmetrical and midline? patency? milia? discharge?

Mouth Inspection and Palpation

Lips: Symmetrical? *thin upper lip?*
Palates: Hard palate—intact? soft palate—intact?
Mucous membrane: Dry? pink? *cyanosis? pale? thrush? Epstein's pearls?*
Sucking reflex: Strong? *weak? uncoordinated? frantic?*
Swallow: Strong? *weak? uncoordinated?*
Tongue: Movement: *protrusion? retrusion? coating?* size and integrity: *hypertrophied?*
Uvula: Intact? midline? *bifid?*

Neck Inspection and Palpation

Movement: Full ROM? *head lag?* limited ROM?
Symmetry: *Webbing? multiple skin folds?*
Masses: *Above or lateral to clavicle?*
Trachea: Midline?
Enlarged thyroid? *None palpated?*

Chest Inspection, Palpation, and Auscultation

Symmetry and proportion: Barrel chest? *supernumerary nipples? breast discharge? breast engorgement?*
Clavicles: Straight? smooth? *crepitus R or L?*
Respirations: Rate? rhythm? thoracic or abdominal breathing? *retractions? grunting? nasal flaring? seesaw respirations?*
Breath sounds: Equal? clear? *rales? rhonchi?*

Heart and Peripheral Vascular Inspection, Palpation, and Auscultation

Heart: Rate? rhythm? murmurs? PMI? S1? S2?
Peripheral pulses: Present, bilateral, symmetrical? (brachial, radial, femoral, popliteal, dorsalis pedis?)
Precordium: *Movement?*

Abdomen Inspection, Auscultation, Palpation, and Percussion

Shape and symmetry: Rounded? symmetrical? *flat? protuberant? scaphoid? asymmetrical? distended?*
Muscle tone: Soft? *flabby and wrinkled? hard and rigid?*
Bowel sounds: Present in all four quadrants? *absent?*
Umbilical stump: Drying? *redness? discharge? bleeding?*
Umbilical vessels: 2 or 3? *meconium staining (see before dye applied)? hernia?*
Bladder distention: Absent? *present?*

Genitalia/Genitourinary Inspection and Palpation

Female: Labia? position of meatus? *vaginal discharge? hymenal tag? size of labia majora versus minora?*
Male: Penis—position of meatus? circumcision? urination within 24 hours? *epispadias? hypospadias? scrotum enlarged? hydrocele? testicles descended? scrotumrugae?*
Anus: Location? patency? meconium?
Buttocks: *Edema or bruising of buttocks?*

Spine Inspection and Palpation

Closed vertebral column? alignment in prone position? incurvation of trunk? Mongolian spot? *pilonidal dimple/sinus? tuft of hair? asymmetry? mass?*

Hips Inspection and Palpation

Symmetrical or *asymmetrical* gluteal fold? *abduction angle? knee-hip length equal? Ortolani maneuver done—any click felt?*

Musculoskeletal Inspection and Palpation

Hands and Feet: Number of digits? ROM? <u>*presence of creases? 1/3, 2/3 or complete surface of soles and palms w/creases? scarf sign? square window? arm recoil? heel to ear flexion?*</u>

Arms and Legs: ROM? flexion? symmetry? equal movements? *positional deformities?*

Neurologic Inspection and Palpation

Reflexes: Hands-grasp reflex? planter reflex? Babinski reflex? stepping reflex? Moro reflex? tonic neck?

Tone: Normal flexion? *flaccidity? spasticity?*

Cry: Normal? no cry, alert and quiet? *weak? shrill? hoarse?*

Behavioral (Observation)

Activity: Active? active with stimulation? quiet? sleeping? baby quiets to soothing, cuddling, or wrapping? *lethargic? irritable? tremors? excessive crying? fretfulness? unable to quiet self?*

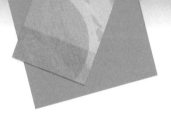

Glossary

A "P" following a term or an abbreviation signifies that it is particularly pertinent in pediatric assessment. A "G" following a term or an abbreviation means that it is particularly pertinent in geriatric assessment.

Accommodation: The ability of the eyes to adapt to viewing objects at various distances

Acrochordons [G]: Skin tags

Acrocyanosis [P]: Blueness (cyanosis) of the newborn's hands and feet caused by slow peripheral perfusion

AC: Air conduction

ADL: Activity of daily living

Adventitious: Abnormal breath sounds

AFDC: Aid to Families with Dependent Children

AK: Above the knee

Alopecia: Loss of hair on head

Ankyloglossia [P]: Tongue-tie

A/P: Anterior/posterior

Apgar score: Screening tool for newborn at birth

Arcus senilis [G]: An opaque white ring around the periphery of the cornea (not pathologic)

Ascites: Serous fluid in abdominal cavity

AV: Arteriovenous

B/A: Bone/air in Rinne hearing test

Barlow's sign: Maneuver to detect subluxation or dislocation of the hip

BC: Bone conduction

Borborygmus: Gurgling, splashing sound over large intestines

BMI: Body mass index

BMR: Basal metabolic rate

BP: Blood pressure

BS: Bowel sounds

BSC: Bedside commode

BSE: Breast self-examination

Brudzinski's sign [P]: Flexion of hips when neck is flexed from supine position

Bruits: Vascular sounds similar to heart murmurs that may be auscultated in areas such as the carotid artery, temple, and epigastrium

Capillary hemangioma [P]: A congenital lesion consisting of numerous closely packed capillaries separated by a network of cells

Caput succedaneum [P]: An edematous swelling of the scalp caused by pressure

CC: Chief complaint, reason that patient is presenting for care or examination

Cephalhematoma [P]: A subperiosteal hemorrhage caused by birth trauma; does not cross suture lines

Cerumen: Earwax

Chloasma: Hyperpigmentation, especially of face, commonly associated with pregnancy

Clubbing: Abnormal enlargement of the distal ends of the fingers and toes, together with curvature of the nails

CN: Cranial nerve

CN I: Olfactory nerve

CN II: Optic nerve

CN III: Oculomotor nerve

CN IV: Trochlear nerve

CN V: Trigeminal nerve

CN VI: Abducens nerve

CN VII: Facial nerve

CN VIII: Acoustic nerve

CN IX: Glossopharyngeal nerve

CN X: Vagus nerve

CN XI: Spinal accessory nerve

CN XII: Hypoglossal nerve

Coloboma: A defect of the pupil of the eye (keyhole pupil)

Comedones [P]: Blackheads

Consanguinity: Related by blood

Consensual constriction: A reflex action whereby a light beam directed into one eye causes not only the pupil of that eye but also that of the other eye to constrict

Crepitus: Crackling noise similar to rubbing hair between fingers

CTA: Clear to auscultation

CT scan: Computed tomography scan

C-V: Cardiovascular

CVA: Cerebrovascular accident; stroke

Cx: Cervix

CXR: Chest x-ray

Cyanosis: Blue-gray color of skin

D and C: Dilatation and curettage

DC: Discontinue

Denver II: Developmental screening tool for children to age 6

DES: Diethylstilbestrol

Diastasis recti: Lateral separation of the two halves of the musculus rectum dominis

DOB: Date of birth

DTRs: Deep tendon reflexes

Dx: Diagnosis

Dyspnea: Difficulty breathing

Dysuria: Difficult painful urination

ECG: Electrocardiogram

Ectropion: Eversion of the edge of an eyelid

EDC: Expected date of confinement

Edema: Swelling

Encopresis: Involuntary discharge of watery feces associated with constipation and fecal retention

ENT: Ear, nose, and throat

Entropion: Inversion of the edge of an eyelid

Enuresis: Involuntary discharge of urine

EOM: Extraocular movement

Epistaxis: Nosebleed

Epstein's pearls [P]: White-yellow accumulation of epithelial cells on hard palate of newborn

Erythema: Diffused redness of skin.

Erythema toxicum neonatorum [P]: A common rash in newborns, characterized by papules or pustules on an erythematous base

Excursion (respiratory): Extent of movement of the diaphragm

Exophthalmos: Abnormal protrusion of eyeball

Exudate: Accumulation of fluid, pus, or serum or matter that penetrates through vessel wall

FHT: Fetal heart tone

Fremitus: A vibration palpated or auscultated through the chest wall

G (for gravid): Pregnant

Gastroschisis [P]: Congenital opening in the wall of the abdomen

Genu valgum: Knock-knee

Genu varum: Bowleg

Gravity: The number of pregnancies

Harlequin sign [P]: A transient redness on one side of the body and paleness on the other; cause unknown

HIV: Human immunodeficiency virus

Hirsutism: Excessive growth of hair in unusual places

Hordeolum: Inflammation of a sebaceous gland of the eyelid

Hx: History

Hypertelorism: Abnormal width between two organs, for example, eyes

Hypertropia: Abnormal turning of eyes upward

Hypotropia: Abnormal turning of eyes downward

IADL: Instrumental activity of daily living

IBW: Ideal body weight

ICS: Intercostal space

Jaundice [P]: Yellowing of the skin; physiologic jaundice; mild jaundice of the newborn caused by functional immaturity of the liver, which results in yellowing after the first 24 hours

JVP: Jugular venous pressure

Kcal: A unit of measure for heat

Keloid: Increased scar formation from previous surgery and/or trauma

Kernig's sign: Reflex contraction and pain in hamstring muscles when extending the leg after flexing the thigh upon the body

Koplik's spots: Small red spots on oral mucosa (sign of measles)

Lanugo [P]: Fine downy hair on the body of infants, especially premature infants

L & W: Living and well

LCM: Left costal margin

Leukoplakia: Formation of white spots or patches on the mucous membrane of the tongue or cheek

Leukorrhea: White or yellow discharge from cervical canal or vagina

LICS: Left intercostal space

LLL: Left lower lobe or left lower leg

LLQ: Left lower quadrant

LMP: Last menstrual period

Lordosis, kyphosis, scoliosis: Swayback, hunchback, lateral curvature of spine

LSB: Left sternal border

LUL: Left upper lobe

LUQ: Left upper quadrant

Macule: See lesion list

MAEW: Moves all extremities well

MCL: Midclavicular line

Menarche: The onset of menses

Metatarsus adductus: Adduction of the forefoot distal to the metatarsal-tarsal line

Milia [P]: Obstructed sebaceous glands, frequently found on the nose and cheeks

Mongolian spot [P]: A bluish black patch over the sacral areas of dark-skinned infants

Montgomery's tubercles: Lubricating glands on nipples

Morphology: The science of structure and form

MRI: Magnetic resonance imaging

MSL: Midsternal line

Nevus flammeus [P]: A circumscribed red, flat lesion found on the face, eyelid, and neck of infants

NG: Nasogastric

Nuchal: Of the neck

Nulliparous: Without births or pregnancies beyond 20 weeks' gestation

Nystagmus: Constant involuntary movement of eyeball

OD: Right eye (Lat., oculo dextro)

Onychomycosis [G]: A fungus infection of the nails, causing thickening, roughness, and splitting

Orthopnea: Breathing easier in erect position

Ortolani test [P]: Test for a congenitally dislocated hip in an infant

OS: Left eye (Lat., oculo sinistro)

OTC: Over the counter (i.e., nonprescription)

OU: Both eyes (Lat., oculi unitas)

Pap: Papanicolaou smear

Paresthesia: Numbness, prickling, tingling

Parity: The state of having borne an infant or infants

Peau d'orange: Dimpled skin condition that resembles the skin of an orange

Pectus carinatum: Abnormal prominence of the sternum

Pectus excavatum: Abnormal depression of the sternum

Peristalsis: Wavelike movements of the alimentary canal

PERRLA: Pupils equal, round, reactive to light, and accommodation

PI: Present illness

Pinna: Auricle or exterior ear

PMI: Point of maximum intensity

Polydactyly: Abnormal number of fingers and toes

Presbycusis [G]: Decreased hearing associated with later maturity

Pseudofolliculitis: Small inflamed pustules near hair follicles caused by shaving too close or short curly hairs that reenter the skin

Ptosis: Drooping of body part (e.g., eyelid)

PVC: Preventricular contraction

Rales: Crackles; added noncontinuous crackling sounds heard on auscultation of the chest; an adventitious sound

RCM: Right costal margin

Rhonchi: Gurgles; added continuous, sonorous, low-pitched sounds heard on auscultation of the chest

Rinne test: A test in which a vibrating tuning fork is used to determine whether a person has normal hearing by comparing the sound perception by bone conduction and by air conduction

RLQ: Right lower quadrant

ROM: Range of motion

RRR: Regular rate and rhythm

RUQ: Right upper quadrant

S_1, S_2, S_3, S_4: Heart sounds

Scaphoid: Boat-shaped, sunken

SIADH: Syndrome of inappropriate antidiuretic hormone

SIDS [P]: Sudden infant death syndrome

Snellen E chart: A wall chart to assess vision

SPF: Skin protection factor for sunscreens and blocks

STD: Sexually transmitted disease

Strabismus: A condition in which the optic axes of the eyes cannot be directed to some object

Striae: Stretch marks, or scarlike breaks in the skin, usually caused by stretching of the skin from weight gain

Syndactyly [P]: Fusion of the toes or fingers

TDD: Telephone device for the deaf

TENS: Transcutaneous electrical nerve stimulation used to relieve pain

Thelarche [P]: Beginning of breast development at puberty

Thrills: Palpable murmur or rub

Tophi: Mineral deposits; tartar

TORCH: Toxoplasmosis, other (viruses), rubella, cytomegalovirus, herpes (simplex viruses)

Torticollis: Head tilts to one side with chin pointing to the other side

Torus palatinus: Benign bony protuberance at the midline of the hard palate

TSE: Testicular self-examination

Turgor: Elasticity of skin

TURP [G]: Transurethral resection of the prostate gland

UTI: Urinary tract infection

Vernix caseosa [P]: A white cheeselike substance found on the skin folds of newborns

Vertigo: Dizziness or lightheadedness

Vesicular: Pertaining to the alveoli of the lungs

Vitiligo: Patches of depigmented skin, piebald skin

W/D: Warm and dry

Weber test for hearing: A test in which a vibrating tuning fork is used to determine which ear is affected by hearing loss

WNL: Within normal limits

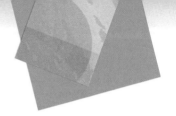

References

Part 1

Agency for Toxic Substances and Disease Registry: Environmental Exposure History. Contact: www.atsdr.cdc.gov, 2001.

Browning, M: Home environment assessment guide. In Hogstel, M (ed): Nursing Care of the Older Adult, ed. 3. Delmar, Albany, NY, 1994, pp 592–595.

Clark, MJ: Community Health Nursing: Caring for Populations, ed. 4. Pearson Education, Upper Saddle River, NJ, 2002.

Folstein, MF, Folstein, SE, and McHugh, PR: Mini-mental state. Journal of Psychiatric Research, 12(1):189–198, 1975.

Friedman, MM: Family Nursing Theory and Practice, ed. 3. McGraw-Hill, New York, 1992.

Hamwi, GJ: Changing Dietary Concepts. In Danowsk, TS (ed): Diabetes Mellitus: Diagnosis and Treatment, Vol 1. American Diabetes Association, Inc, New York, 1964, pp. 73–78.

Hogstel, MO: Assessing mental status. J Geront Nurs 17(5):43, 1991.

Jarvis, C (ed): Physical Examination. WB Saunders, Philadelphia, 2000.

Katz, S, Ford, AB, and Moskowitz, RW, et al: Studies of illness in the aged: The index of ADL. JAMA 185:914–919, 1963.

Kozier, B, Erb, G, Berman, A, and Snyder, SJ (eds): Fundamentals of Nursing, ed. 7. Pearson Prentice Hall, Upper Saddle River, NJ, 2004, p. 485, 614

Mahoney, FI, and Barthel, DW: Functional evaluation: The Barthel index. Maryland Med J 14:61–65, 1965.

National Standards for Culturally and Linguistically Appropriate Services in Health Care. United States Department of Health and Human Services, Office of Minority Health, Washington, DC, March 2001. Prepared under Contract No 282-99-039. IQ Solutions, Rockville, MD.

Partnership for Clear Health Communication (n.d.). What Can Providers Do? Ask Me 3. Retrieved 17 March 2004 from http://www.askme3.org/

Seidel, HM, Ball, JW, Dains, JE, and Benedict GW: Mosby's Guide to Physical Examination, ed. 5. Mosby Year-Book, St. Louis, 2003.

Stanhope, M, and Lancaster, J: Community Health Nursing, ed. 6. Mosby, St Louis, 2004.

US Census, 2000.

Part 2

Kozier, B, Erb, G, Berman, A, and Snyder, SJ (eds): Fundamentals of Nursing, ed. 7. Pearson Prentice Hall, Upper Saddle River, NJ, 2004.

Potter, PA, and Perry, AG: Fundamentals of Nursing, ed. 5. Mosby, St Louis, 2001, pp 730–731.

Part 3

Dash, ME, Foster, EB, Smith, DM, Phillips, SL: Urinary incontinence: The social health maintenance organization's approach (CE). Geriatric Nursing, 25(2):83–85, 2004.

Jarvis, C. (ed): Physical Examination and Health Assessment. WB Saunders, Philadelphia, 2000.

Kozier, B, Erb, G, Berman, A, and Snyder, SJ (eds): Fundamentals of Nursing, ed. 7. Pearson Prentice Hall, Upper Saddle River, NJ, 2004, p. 485.

Merkel, S, Voepel-Lewis, T, and Malviya, S: Pain control, pain assessment in infants and young children: The FLACC scale: A behavioral tool to measure pain in young children. American Journal of Nursing, 102(10):55–56, 58, 2002.

Murray, RB, and Zentner, JP: Nursing Assessment and Health Promotion Strategies Through the Lifespan, ed. 7. Prentice Hall, Upper Saddle River, NJ, 2001, p 51.

Seidel, HM, Ball, JW, Dains, JE, and Benedict, GW: Mosby's Guide to Physical Examination, ed. 5. Mosby, St. Louis, 2003, p. 189.

Seidel, H, Ball, J, and Benedict, GW: Mosby's Physical Examination Handbook, ed 3. Mosby, St Louis, 2003, p 67, p. 98, 99.

Tanner, JM: Foetus into Man: Physical Growth From Conception to Maturity. Harvard University Press, Cambridge, MA, 1990.

U.S. Department of Health and Human Services: Clinical Practice Guideline: Treatment of Pressure Ulcers. USDHHS, Public Health Service, Agency for Health Care Policy and Research, Rockville, MD, December 1994, vol 15.

United States Department of Health and Human Services, National Heart, Lung, and Blood Institute: Seventh Report of the Joint National Committee on the Prevention, Detection, Evaluation, and Treatment of High Blood Pressure. NIH Pub No. 03–5233 (electronic version). National Heart, Lung, Blood Institute Information Center, Bethesda, MD, May 2003, retrieved 17 March 04 from http://www.nhlbi.nih.gov/guidelines/hypertension/express.pdf.

Venes, D & Thomas, C (eds): Taber's Cyclopedic Medical Dictionary, ed 19. FA Davis, Philadelphia, 2001.

Vision Screening Manual, Texas Department of Health, Austin, TX, 1998, p. 22.

Wong, DL, Hockenberry-Eaton, M, Wilson D, Winkelstein, ML, and Schwartz, P: Wong's Essentials of Pediatric Nursing ed. 6, Mosby, St Louis, 2001, p. 1301. www.cdc.gov/chooseyourcover/ganda.htm#when

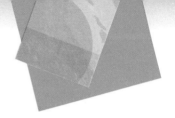

Bibliography

Agency for Toxic Substances and Disease Registry: Environmental Exposure History, Contact: www.atsdr.cdc.gov, 2001.

Average height and weight for persons aged 65 years and older. Morrison's manual of clinical nutrition management. JAMA, 172:165, 1960.

Blackburn, GL, Bistrian, BR: Nutritional and metabolic assessment of the hospitalized patient. JPEN, 1:11, 1977.

Browning, M: Home environment assessment guide. In Hogstel, M (ed): Nursing Care of the Older Adult, ed. 3. Delmar, Albany, NY, 1994, pp. 592–595.

Calonge, N: Screening for obesity in adults: Recommendations and rationale. US Preventive Services Task Force, Washington, DC. American Journal of Nursing, 104(5): 94–101, 2004.

Clark, MJ: Community Health Nursing: Caring for Populations, ed. 4. Pearson Education, Upper Saddle River, NJ, 2002.

Clinical Guidelines for the Identification, Evaluation, and Treatment of Overweight and Obesity in Adults: The Evidence Report. National Heart, Lung, and Blood Institute in cooperation with the National Institute of Diabetes and Digestive and Kidney Diseases, http://www.nhlbi.nih.gov/guidelines/obesity/obhome.htm

Dash, ME, Foster, EB, Smith, DM, Phillips, SL: Urinary incontinence: The social health maintenance organization's approach (CE). Geriatric Nursing, 25(2):81–89, 2004.

Folstein, MF, Folstein, SE, and McHugh, PR: Mini-mental state. Journal of Psychiatric Research, 12(1):189–198, 1975.

Friedman, MM: Family Nursing Theory and Practice, ed. 3. McGraw-Hill, New York, 1992.

Hamwi, GJ: Changing Dietary Concepts. In Danowsk, TS (ed): Diabetes Mellitus: Diagnosis and Treatment, Vol 1. American Diabetes Association, Inc, New York, 1964, pp. 73–78.

Hogstel, M: Gerontology: Nursing Care of the Older Adult. Delmar, New York, 2001.

Hogstel, MO: Assessing mental status. J Geront Nurs, 17(5):43, 1991.

Jarvis, C (ed): Physical Examination and Health Assessment. WB Saunders, Philadelphia, 2000.

Katz, S, Ford, AB, Moskowitz, RW, et al: Studies of illness in the aged: The index of ADL. JAMA, 185:914–919, 1963.

Kozier, B, Erb, G, Berman, A, and Snyder, SJ (eds): Fundamentals of Nursing, ed. 7. Pearson Prentice Hall. Upper Saddle River, NJ, 2004, pp. 485, 614.

Mahoney, FI, and Barthel, DW: Functional evaluation: The Barthel index. Maryland Med J, 14:61–65, 1965.

Merkel, S, Voepel-Lewis, T, and Malviya, S: Pain control, pain assessment in infants and young children: The FLACC scale: A behavioral tool to measure pain in young children. American Journal of Nursing, 102(10):55–56, 58, 2002.

Murray, RB, and Zentner, JP: Nursing Assessment and Health Promotion Strategies Through the Lifespan, ed. 7. Prentice Hall, Upper Saddle River, NJ, 2001, p. 51.

National Standards for Culturally and Linguistically Appropriate Services in Health Care. United States Department of Health and Human Services, Office of Minority Health, Washington, DC, March 2001. Prepared under Contract No 282-99-039. Rockville, MD, IQ Solutions.

National Center for Health Statistics in Collaboration with the National Center for Chronic Diseases Prevention and Health Promotion, 2000, http://www.cdc.gov/growthcharts

New high blood pressure guidelines American Heart Association Fighting Heart Disease, June 3, 2003. http://www.americanheart.org/presenter:jhtml? identifier = 3011728

Nutrition and Your Health: Dietary Guidelines for Americans, ed. 3. Washington, DC: US Department of Agriculture and Health and Human Services 1990 Home and Garden Bulletin No 232.

Partnership for Clear Health Communication (n.d.). What Can Providers Do? Ask Me 3: Retrieved 17 March 2004 from http://www.askme3.org/

Potter, PA, and Perry, AG: Fundamentals of Nursing, ed. 5. Mosby, St Louis, 2001, pp. 730–731.

Practical Guide: Identification, Evaluation and Treatment of Overweight and Obesity in Older Adults; developed by the North American Association for the Study of Obesity (NAASO) and the National Heart, Lung, and Blood Institute (NHLBI 2000), http://www.nhlbi.nih.gov/guidelines/obesity/practgde.htm

Report of the Dietary Guidelines Advisory Committee on the Dietary Guidelines for Americans, 2000, p. 3, http://www.usda.gov/cnpp/Pubs/DG2000/

Rosenbam, JG, FACS, Cleveland, OH.

Seidel, H, Ball, J, and Benedict, GW: Mosby's Physical Examination Handbook, ed. 3. Mosby, St Louis, 2003.

Seidel, HM, Ball JW, Dains, JE, and Benedict, GW: Mosby's Guide to Physical Examination, ed. 3. Mosby-Year Book, St Louis, 2003, p. 67.

Stanhope, M, Lancaster, J: Community Health Nursing, ed. 6. Mosby, St Louis, 2004.

Tanner, JM: Fetus into Man: Physical Growth From Conception to Maturity. Harvard University Press, Cambridge, MA, 1990.

United States Department of Health and Human Services, National Heart, Lung, and Blood Institute: Seventh Report of the Joint National Committee on the Prevention, Detection, Evaluation, and Treatment of High Blood Pressure. NIH Pub No. 03-5233 (electronic version). National Heart, Lung, and Blood Institute Information Center, Bethesda, MD, May 2003, retrieved March 17, 2004, from http://www. nhlbi.nih. gov/guidelines/hypertension/express.pdf.

U.S. Department of Health and Human Services: Clinical Practice Guidelines: Treatment of Pressure Ulcers. USDHHS, Public Health Service, Agency for Health Care Policy and Research, Rockville, MD, December 1994, vol 15.

U.S. Department of Health and Human Services: The Clinician's Handbook of Preventive Services. USDHHS, Alexandria, VA, 1994.

Venes, D and Thomas, C (eds): Taber's Cyclopedic Medical

Dictionary, ed. 19. FA Davis, Philadelphia, 2001, pp. 815, 2196.

Vision Screening Manual, Texas Department of Health, Austin, TX, 1998, p. 22.

Wong, DL, Hockenberry-Eaton, M, Wilson, D, Winkelstein, ML, and Schwartz, P: Wong's Essentials of Pediatric Nursing, Rd. 6 Mosby, St Louis, Mo, 2001, p. 1301 www.cdc.gov/chooseyourcover/qanda.htm#when

INDEX

Note: Page numbers followed by the letter f refer to figures; page numbers followed by the letter t refer to tables.